T0211283

Lecture Notes in Computer Science 9062

Commenced Publication in 1973
Founding and Former Series Editors:
Gerhard Goos, Juris Hartmanis, and Jan van Leeuwen

Editorial Board

More information about this series at http://www.springer.com/series/7408

Michaela Huhn · Laurie Williams (Eds.)

Software Engineering in Health Care

4th International Symposium, FHIES 2014
and 6th International Workshop, SEHC 2014
Washington, DC, USA, July 17–18, 2014
Revised Selected Papers

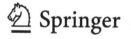 Springer

Editors
Michaela Huhn
TU Clausthal
Clausthal-Zellerfeld
Germany

Laurie Williams
North Carolina State University
Raleigh, NC
USA

ISSN 0302-9743   ISSN 1611-3349   (electronic)
Lecture Notes in Computer Science
ISBN 978-3-319-63193-6   ISBN 978-3-319-63194-3   (eBook)
DOI 10.1007/978-3-319-63194-3

Library of Congress Control Number: 2017946686

LNCS Sublibrary: SL2 – Programming and Software Engineering

Printed on acid-free paper

This Springer imprint is published by Springer Nature
The registered company is Springer International Publishing AG
The registered company address is: Gewerbestrasse 11, 6330 Cham, Switzerland

Preface

This proceedings volume documents the joint event of the 4th Symposium on Foundations of Health Information Engineering and Systems (FHIES) and the Software Engineering in Healthcare (SEHC) workshop held during July 17–18, 2014, in Washington DC. The goal of FHIES/SEHC 2014 was to discuss recent research innovations and to integrate an interdisciplinary community to develop a research, educational, and industrial agenda for the application of software engineering in the health-care sector.

The ability to deliver timely, effective, and cost-efficient health-care services remains one of the world's foremost challenges. The challenge has numerous dimensions including: (a) the need to develop a highly functional yet secure electronic health record system that integrates a multitude of incompatible existing systems; (b) in-home patient support systems and telemedicine to reduce demand on professional health-care facilities; (c) innovative technical devices, such as advanced pacemakers that support other health-care procedures; and (d) the specific constraints for health care imposed in different societies, particularly developing countries. Responding to this challenge will substantially increase the usage of software-intensive systems in all aspects of health-care services. However, the digitization of health care results in extensive changes related to the development, use, evolution, and integration of health software, especially with respect to the volume, dependability, safety, and security of these software-dependent systems.

The call for submissions attracted 23 submissions from around the world in a number of the areas mentioned in the call for papers. After the usual and thorough peer-review process (papers were reviewed by three or four members of the Program Committee), 16 papers were accepted for presentation in the proceedings of the workshop. The current version of the papers reflect additional feedback given to the authors through additional post-conference paper reviews and conversations that took place at the conference.

The papers cover a range of relevant and interesting topics. There are several papers on security aspects of health information systems. Another set of papers deal with medical devices in cyberphysical systems. Other papers focus on the process of providing health care and monitoring patients. Finally, several papers focus on patient safety and the assurance of medical systems.

The organizers would like to thank our sponsors for their support throughout this venture: TU Clausthal, McMaster Centre for Software Certification, and the Software Engineering Institute. Thanks to the general chairs, Wendy MacCaull (St. Francis Xavier University, Canada), Kevin Sullivan (University of Virginia, USA), and Alan Wassyng (McMaster University, Canada), and the hard-working members of the Program Committee and their additional reviewers. We appreciate the support of EasyChair for the paper review process and to generate these proceedings.

July 2014

Michaela Huhn
Laurie Williams

Organization

Program Committee

Elske Ammenwerth	UMIT
George Avrunin	University of Massachusetts, USA
Ruth Breu	Research Group Quality Engineering
Tom Broens	MobiHealth B.V.
Lori Clarke	UMass Amherst, USA
Jeremy Gibbons	University of Oxford, UK
Mats Heimdahl	University of Minnesota, USA
Jozef Hooman	Embedded Systems Institute and Radboud University Nijmegen, The Netherlands
Michaela Huhn	Technische Universität Clausthal, Institut für Informatik, Germany
Craig Kuziemsky	University of Ottawa, Canada
Brian R. Larson	Kansas State University, USA
Yves Ledru	Laboratoire d'Informatique de Grenoble - Université Joseph Fourier, France
Insup Lee	University of Pennsylvania, USA
Martin Leucker	University of Lübeck, Germany
Zhiming Liu	Birmingham City University, UK
Orlando Loques	Universidade Federal Fluminense, Brazil
Brad Malin	Vanderbilt University, USA
Dominique Mery	Université de Lorraine, LORIA, France
Deshendran Moodley	University of KwaZulu-Natal, South Africa
Leon Osterweil	UMass Amherst, USA
Barbara Paech	Universität Heidelberg, Germany
Liam Peyton	University of Ottawa, Canada
Andy Podgurski	Case Western Reserve University, USA
Jetley Raoul	ABB
Joachim Reiss	
Ita Richardson	Lero - Irish Software Engineering Research Centre, University of Limerick, Ireland
Kamran Sartipi	University of Ontario Institute of Technology, Canada
Bernhard Schätz	TU München, Germany
Eleni Stroulia	University of Alberta, Canada
Kevin Sullivan	University of Virginia, USA
Alan Wassyng	McMaster University, Canada
Jens Weber	University of Victoria, Canada
Charles Weinstock	Software Engineering Institute
Laurie Williams	North Carolina State University, USA
Yi Zhang	US FDA, USA

Additional Reviewers

Boehm, Thomas
Chiarabini, Luca
Roederer, Alex
Sauerwein, Clemens
Schmitz, Malte

Sillaber, Christian
Sulieman, Lina
Wang, Shaohui
Zhang, Wen

Contents

Patient Flow Monitoring Systems: Investigation of Alternatives

Omar Badreddin[1(✉)] and Liam Peyton[2]

[1] Department of Computer Science, University of Texas, El Paso, USA
obbadreddin@utep.edu
[2] School of Electrical Engineering and Computer Science, University of Ottawa, Ottawa, Canada
lpeyton@uottawa.ca

Abstract. Hospitals need to reduce wait times in emergency rooms to ensure timely delivery of services. This paper provides an in-depth investigation and evaluation of three distinct approaches to provide real time monitoring of patient flow. The three approaches differ in the number and nature of their data sources. The results suggest that additional data sources provide only little improvements in the monitoring capabilities. Monitoring patient flow can be achieved in real time with potentially little need for expensive and complex integration with hospital information systems by collecting location data or by using data collected from electronic forms.

Keywords: Real time patient flow management system · Business process management · Wait time · Business intelligence · Complex event processing

1 Introduction

Analysis of patients wait times is an activity typically performed by hospitals, long after a service has been delivered to patients. Analysis of wait times in real time has remained elusive to date. This is because the existing healthcare systems are fragmented and are not developed to address such a real-time requirement. In addition, the data logged in the existing healthcare systems are sometimes inaccurate as data entry may take place hours or even days after it is initially recorded on paper.

A number of approaches have emerged to address real time monitoring of patients flow. In the first approach, location data is collected and integrated with the existing hospital information systems to infer key patient states [1]. Once the states have been inferred, real time dashboards can report on patient progress along the clinical pathways in real time. The second approach is a forms-only approach, which collects data from existing electronic clinical forms to monitor patient flow [2]. The third approach, we refer to here as location only approach, relies on the analysis of the location data of both patients and clinicians to infer patients states and flow. This approach does not involve hospital information systems or electronic forms, and relies exclusively on location data [3].

Each of these approaches represents a distinctive paradigm. The first approach attempts to achieve the most comprehensive monitoring, while at the same time

© Springer International Publishing AG 2017
M. Huhn and L. Williams (Eds.): FHIES 2014/SEHC 2014, LNCS 9062, pp. 1–9, 2017.
DOI: 10.1007/978-3-319-63194-3_1

minimizing any overhead to clinicians. This approach maximizes monitoring potential by correlating data from multiple sources. The down side is complexity and cost. Such an approach requires integration with hospital information systems and triangulation of location data with care operational data. The forms approach attempts to use electronic forms to collect operational data to report on patients flow. In most cases, new mobile apps have to be built to provide adequate monitoring support in real-time. The location-only approach utilizes location tags that track location and movements data. This approach attempts to avoid the costly integration with hospital information systems while providing adequate levels of flow monitoring.

This paper is organized as follows. Background and significance of the work is discussed, followed by a presentation of related work. The ACS clinical pathway is introduced as a reference clinical pathway for the empirical evaluation. We then introduce the empirical evaluation of the three approaches. The limitations of the work are then discussed. We conclude the paper in Sect. 9.

2   Related Work

The value of workflow management tools and Business Process Management (BPM) technology is well identified and documented [15]. Becker et al. [11] has reported their work on using BPM technology to help coordinate disparate data sources in a large urban hospital in the U.S. Their work highlights the potential of BPM in supporting and automating clinical decisions. Hajo et al. [12] has deployed BPM technology to demonstrate flexible support for clinical pathways. Their approach relies on identifying 'flexible patterns' to accommodate the unpredictability of clinical processes.

Manfred [13] has articulated the unpredictability of clinical processes, and provides an analysis of recent BPM advancements that can better address some of this unpredictability. Specifically, Manfred identifies improvements in process adaptation, flexibility, and evolution.

Zhu et al. [4] has developed real time monitoring dashboards for a Radiology department in the central hospital in China. They relied exclusively on integration with existing hospital systems and BPM. They are able to monitor key states and patient flows. They did not include any location information, and hence, the identified states are at a high level. For example, this approach is not able to calculate how long the patient has been waiting inside the MRI room.

Yao et al. [5] proposed complex event processing to be used along with RFID technology to improve patient safety and procedural efficiencies for surgical procedures. They are able to infer key states for the identified surgical clinical pathway using location data alone. This is largely because in this clinical pathway, the patient is transported from room to room as they progress through the clinical pathway. Therefore, tracking the location of the patient is sufficient to infer the patient progress along the clinical pathway.

Long running care processes, those that can span months and years, can be sufficiently monitored using traditional forms applications [2]. This is because accuracy within a few days is typically sufficient. For example, typical operational guidelines may require that a referral be scheduled within 48 h, and the patient appointment be within 14 days of referral. Such level of granularity may be sufficiently achieved using forms applications.

3 Background and Significance

In Canada, as well as in many parts of the world, healthcare organizations face challenges with patient wait times, particularly in Emergency Departments (ED). By their nature, EDs face fluctuating and unpredictable inflows of patients, many of whom require immediate attention. According to a study by the Canadian Institute for Health Information (CIHI) [6], a significant majority of patients whose condition requires urgent care end up in the ED. Ontario Ministry of Health made its top-priority health concern to address the wait time issue by launching "The Ontario Wait Times Strategy Program" which commenced in 2008. This program requires hospitals to report on patients wait times, and to facilitate access to key procedures and services, such as X-rays and MRIs.

A study of wait times at EDs [7] reveals significant unpredictability and variability in patient wait times. Achieving medical targets also exhibited significant variability. The study also finds that longer wait times for admission is highly correlated with longer visit duration. Another study has found high positive correlation between wait times, mortality and readmission rate [8]. The study reports that patients arriving at ED during shifts with longer wait times are more likely to be admitted to the hospital, even though they may be well enough to leave the hospital on the same day.

Despite the significant potential in monitoring patient flow, identifying bottlenecks, and discovering root causes, basic patient flow monitoring remains absent from most care institutions [9, 10].

4 Reference Clinical Pathway

A detailed process model that documents the Acute Coronary Syndrome (ACS) clinical pathway at a large community hospital in Ontario has been developed [16]. The process model of the ACS clinical pathway details all the steps and tasks performed by every participating clinician. It also documents system interactions, medical forms, medical guidelines and best practices. This was achieved by shadowing all participating clinicians as they handle patients walking into the ED with a chest pain, and who are later diagnosed as ACS patients. The models and documentation were verified and validated by hospital staff.

The ACS process starts at patient triage, and ends at discharge. The process includes multiple patient assessments, blood tests, patient transportation to different hospital units. Table 1 summarizes only the key clinical pathway states. The complete ACS clinical pathway is published in another work [16].

Table 1. Detailed patient states along the ACS clinical pathway

	State name	Start	End
1	Triaged	Patient info entered in system, location tag assigned.	The nurse completes the triage and takes the patient to the waiting room.
2	Waiting for initial assessment	Triage ended.	Physician walks into the room and starts examining the patient.
3	In initial assessment	Waiting for initial assessment state ended.	Physician leaves room after examination and submits initial assessment form.
4	Waiting for lab results	Blood work is requested.	The lab sends back results.
5	Waiting for reassessment	Lab results have arrived.	Physician walks into the room and starts re-examining the patient.
6	In re-assessment	Waiting for reassessment has ended.	Physician completes re-examination, requests bed for patient.
7	Waiting for bed	In re-assessment ended.	A bed is available for the patient.
8	Waiting for transport	Transport is requested.	Transport personnel arrives.

5   Evaluation of Patient Flow Monitoring Approaches

We have developed three different implementations of the reference clinical pathway corresponding to each approach. The first implementation uses location data, and data coming from a simulation of the hospital information system. We refer to this implementation as *'combined approach'*. The second implementation, the *'forms only approach'*, implements the clinical pathway using forms application without using any location data. The forms are developed to mimic the hospital existing forms, with modifications and additions that compensates for the missing data required for the real time reporting. The third implementation utilizes location tags that are assigned to each participant in the clinical pathway, including the patient, nurses, physicians, transport and housekeeping personnel. We refer to this approach as *'location only approach'*.

5.1   Simulation Exercises

The *'combined approach'* was validated through a series of walk-through evaluations at the premises of a large urban hospital in Canada [16]. The walk-through evaluations took place in a section of the hospital that was not being used. Clinicians from the hospital participated. Clinicians had the choice to participate as patients, clinicians or staff. The walk-through evaluation did not include real patients and assumed zero variability. The walk-through evaluation included a simulation of the hospital electronic healthcare records (EHR). For example, when a lab test is requested, the lab and its tests results were simulated. No actual samples were taken or tested during the walk-through evaluation.

Once the *'combined approach'* was validated, we conducted a thorough analysis of all three implementations in a simulation exercise back at our university research lab. The lab space was divided up into several rooms and sections. The mapping included operating rooms, patients' rooms and beds. Open space was also utilized to represent similar open areas where patients arrive and wait for admission. For this exercise, the location tags were calibrated to use the existing Wi-Fi signal for open spaces. When high precision was required, we utilized infrared signals and beacons that were mounted on the walls. This simulation was conducted using student participants who played the roles of patients, clinicians, transport, and housekeeping. The goal of the simulation was to verify and compare the technologies in use. Our focus was on ensuring that locations and progress through the clinical pathway was being tracked effectively with reasonable delays and accuracy.

6 Evaluation Criteria

We evaluate the three implementations using the following three criteria.

1. Coverage of real time monitoring of patient states

This is measured by the number of states whose start and end can be identified. For example, the state number 4 in Table 1 *'waiting for test results'* starts when the test have been requested and ends when the results are sent back from the lab. In the same table, state number 6 *'In reassessment'* starts when the patient is waiting for reassessment by a physician after the test results has been received, and ends when the physician starts to reassess the patient. Table 2 below summarizes this evaluation criterion for these two states.

Table 2. State identification using the three paradigms

Approach		Waiting for Test results	In reassessment
Combined	Start	Form	Form and Location
	End	EHR	Form and Location
Forms only	Start	Form	Form
	End	N/A	Form
Location only	Start	N/A	Location
	End	N/A	Location

The evaluation criteria did not include reliability. For example, a physician may start examining the patient before he opens the reassessment form. In this case, the actual start of the state identification is inaccurate in the case of forms only system. Similarly, for the location only system, a physician may walk into the room for reasons other than examining the patient. This may result in unreliable data in the system, but for the purposes of this evaluation, it was not taken into consideration as it was hard to quantify. We assumed that all participants behaved in the same systematic manner.

2. Overhead to clinicians

This is measured by the number of additional forms and clicks that are required in order to identify the start and end of the patient states, as compared to the hospital existing system. Here, we distinguish between clicks and forms; additional clicks are required on *existing forms*. In other words, a new click is required to be added on a form that already exists in the current hospital system. The click is required to identify the beginning or end of a patient's state. In other cases, a new click is required at a time where there is no existing form in place at the current system.

The distinction is important for two reasons. Both, a new click and a new form represent an overhead to clinicians. However, a new click means that the overhead is minimal, as the clinician is already interacting with the system. On the other hand, a new form poses additional overhead for clinicians who may need to access the system at a time where they do not typically do. A new form also represents additional development effort to integrate the new form into the system.

3. Complexity

This is measured by the number of integration points; i.e., the number of data sources that are required to support the implementation. In the case of the combined approach, the data sources are events from the existing health care system, location data, and forms data. In the case of forms only and location only approaches, there is only a single data source, forms and location data respectively.

The complexity associated with the integration points depends on the number and nature of the data sources involved. For example, if a system involves three integration points from the same source system, then this would be less complex if the three distinct systems involved. We do not take the nature of the integration points into consideration in this study.

7 Results and Analysis

The results of our analysis of the reference clinical pathway are summarized in Table 3.

Table 3. Summary of analysis results

Approach	Identifiable start states	Identifiable end state	Identifiable start and end states
Combined	23	23	23 (100%)
Forms only (no extra clicks)	15	13	10 (43.5%)
Forms only (with extra clicks[1])	23	23	23 (100%)
Location only	15	19	14 (61%)

1 Additional clicks are estimated to be 18 clicks and 13 new forms within the ACS clinical pathway.

As shown in the table above, the combined approach is able to identify 100% of all start and end states. This is because this approach triangulates data from multiple sources to identify these states. On the other hand, using the forms only, the system is able to identify 43.5% of all start and end states. However, if we add 18 clicks and 13 new forms, we can compensate for the missing data sources to identify 100% of all start and end states. The third paradigm, the location only approach, can identify 61% of all starts and ends for all states.

These results highlight the potential of using the existing forms application to monitor patients flow. Theoretically, about 50% monitoring can be achieved without investing in additional infrastructure to track location or integrate with EHRs. In addition, 29% of the state boundaries identified are bed related, and 16.6% are transportation related. If we were to exclude these two categories of states, then the monitoring potential increases to 70%.

8   Threats to Validity

Our study of the three approaches faces a couple of threats to validity. The effectiveness of the treatment in the ACS clinical pathway is time sensitive. The sooner a diagnosis can be established, the sooner the operation can be performed, the better the outcome. Studies show that delay beyond 90 min means that an operation may not be as effective as other secondary treatment options. This clinical pathway may not be a good representation for other clinical pathways. Therefore, one must be careful at generalizing the results to other clinical pathways.

There is an external validity threat that the forms in use at the targeted hospital may not be a good representation of how other hospitals implement the same clinical pathway. At the community hospital where the study was conducted, there was almost no paper trail and all forms were electronic. The results of this study may reveal different results in hospitals where a significant portion of the process is only documented on paper and not online. In addition, other hospitals may implement a variation of the ACS clinical pathway that may result in different patient states.

Finally, our estimate of the cost and complexity is based on the number of data sources and the number of extra clicks and new forms. This measure may not be a good representation of the actual complexity or cost.

9   Conclusion

Monitoring patient flow is a growing trend in urban hospitals for multiple reasons. Acute Coronary Syndrome (ACS) falls under the category of care services that must be delivered in timely manner. Hospitals struggle to meet their medical and regulatory guidelines for care delivery and patient wait times. When excessive delays occur, it is difficult for hospitals to identify the root cause of delays.

This paper evaluated three approaches for real time monitoring of patients wait times based on the ACS clinical pathway. Our analysis suggests that the combined approach is able to monitor all patient states without requiring additional burden to care givers. This is achieved at the cost of system complexity. A system that combines data from multiple sources is both complex and expensive. The forms only paradigm can monitor about half of patient states using only the existing medical electronic forms. Location only can monitor about 60% of patient states.

The wide variety of clinical pathways may result in different paradigm being more suitable for different group of pathways. Long term clinical pathways may be best suited for forms only paradigms, emergency and time critical processes may benefit from the combined paradigm. This variety of clinical pathways suggests that a study be performed to categorize the different type of clinical pathways in terms of their monitoring requirements.

References

1. Behnam, S.A., Badreddin, O.: Toward a care process metamodel. In: ICSE Workshop on Software Engineering in Health Care (2013)
2. Kuziemsky, C.E., Weber-Jahnke, J.H., Lau, F., Downing, G.M.: An interdisciplinary computer based information tool for palliative severe pain management. J. Am. Med. Inf. Assoc. 15(3), 374–382 (2008)
3. Lenert, L.A., et al.: Design and evaluation of a wireless electronic health records system for field care in mass casualty settings. J. Am. Med. Inf. Assoc. 18(6), 842–852 (2011)
4. Zhu, Q., et al.: Radiology workflow-based monitor-ing dashboard in a heterogeneous environment. In: 2010 3rd International Conference on Biomedical Engineering and Informatics (BMEI), vol. 6. IEEE (2010)
5. Yao, W., Chu, C.-H., Li, Z.: Leverag-ing complex event processing for smart hospitals us-ing RFID. J. Netw. Comput. Appl. 34(3), 799–810 (2011)
6. Canadian Institute for Health Information (CIHI).: Who is using emergency depart-ments and how long are they waiting? CIHI Website (2005). ISBN: 1-55392-676-5
7. Horwitz, L.I., Green, J., Bradley, E.H.: US emergency department performance on wait time and length of visit. Ann. Emer. Med. 55(2), 133–141 (2010)
8. Guttmann, A., et al.: Association between waiting times and short term mortality and hospital admission after departure from emergency department: population based cohort study from Ontario, Canada. BMJ: Br. Med. J. 342 (2011)
9. Gupta, D., Denton, B.: Appointment scheduling in health care: challenges and opportunities. IIE Trans. 40(9), 800–819 (2008)
10. Patrick, J., Puterman, M.L.: Reducing wait times through operations research: Optimizing the use of surge capacity. Healthc. Pol. 3(3), 75–88 (2008)
11. Becker, J., Fischer, R., Janiesch, C.: ERCIS Münster. optimizing US health care processes-a case study in business process management. In: AMCIS (2007)
12. Reijers, H.A., Russell, N., van der Geer, S., Krekels, G.A.M.: Workflow for healthcare: a methodology for realizing flexible medical treatment processes. In: Rinderle-Ma, S., Sadiq, S., Leymann, F. (eds.) Business Process Management Workshops, BPM 2009. LNBIP, vol. 43, pp. 593–604. Springer, Berlin (2010)
13. Reichert, M.: What BPM technology can do for healthcare process support. In: Peleg, M., Lavrač, N., Combi, C. (eds.) AIME 2011. LNCS, vol. 6747, pp. 2–13. Springer, Heidelberg (2011). doi:10.1007/978-3-642-22218-4_2
14. Lenz, R., Reichert, M.: IT support for healthcare processes–premises, challenges, perspectives. Data Knowl. Eng. 61(1), 39–58 (2007)

15. Pourshahid, A., Peyton, L., Ghanavati, S., Amyot, D., Chen, P., Weiss, M.: Model-based validation of business processes. In: Shankararaman, V., Zhao, J.L., Lee, J.K. (eds.) Business Enterprise, Process, and Technology Management: Models and Applications, Business Science Reference, pp. 165–183. IGI Global, Hershey (2012). doi: 10.4018/978-1-46660-249-6
16. Tchemeube, R.B., Amyot, D., Mouttham, A.: Location-aware business process management for real-time monitoring of a cardiac care process. In: CASCON 2013 Proceedings of the 2013 Conference of the Center for Advanced Studies on Collaborative Research, Toronto, Canada, pp. 230–244. IBM Corp., Riverton, November 2013

Retrofitting Communication Security into a Publish/Subscribe Middleware Platform

Carlos Salazar and Eugene Y. Vasserman$^{(\boxtimes)}$

Kansas State University, Manhattan, USA
{csalazar,eyv}@ksu.edu

Abstract. The Medical Device Coordination Framework (MDCF) is an open source middleware package for interoperable medical devices, designed to support the emerging Integrated Clinical Environment (ICE) interoperability standard. As in any open system, medical devices connected to the MDCF or other ICE-like network should be authenticated to defend the system against malicious, dangerous, or otherwise unauthorized devices. In this paper, we describe the creation and integration of a pluggable, flexible authentication system into the almost 18,000 lines of MDCF codebase, and evaluate the performance of proof-of-concept device authentication providers. The framework is sufficiently expressive to support arbitrary modules implementing arbitrary authentication protocols using arbitrarily many rounds of communication. In contrast with the expected costs in securing nontrivial systems, often involving major architectural changes and significant degradation of system performance, our solution requires the addition of just over 1,000 lines of code ($\sim 5.56\%$), and incurs performance overhead only from the authentication protocols themselves, rather than from the framework.

1 Introduction

Medical devices have a history of being stand-alone units [1,2], and most devices currently used in clinical environments stay true to this paradigm. Even when a device manufacturer has implemented some interoperability features, they are not designed to interoperate with devices or software from other manufacturers. Interoperability is confined to vertically integrated systems, preventing technology diversification and promoting vendor lock-in. When implemented, connectivity is typically only used for logging device data [1]. Simply put, medical devices do not play well with others. This stands in contrast to other domains such as avionics, which implement cross-vendor interoperability using an integrated platform [3].

Many in the clinical and medical device community see a need for an integrated "system of systems" for medical devices. This has led to the creation of the Integrated Clinical Environment (ICE) standard [4] and the Medical Device Coordination Framework (MDCF) project [5]. MDCF is a publish/subscribe middleware for coordinating medical devices, architected in logical units analogous to those described in the ICE standard.

© Springer International Publishing AG 2017
M. Huhn and L. Williams (Eds.): FHIES 2014/SEHC 2014, LNCS 9062, pp. 10–25, 2017.
DOI: 10.1007/978-3-319-63194-3_2

While interoperable medical systems can provide numerous benefits, such as improved patient safety, reduced medical errors, and automated clinical workflows [5,6], there are serious security and privacy concerns given the sensitive nature of patients' medical data. An attacker who could alter data or prevent its transmission could cause serious harm, or even death. Consequently, authentication, encryption, and more advanced data protection features must be incorporated into the MDCF. These functions should be implemented in a modular manner, allowing device manufacturers to implement as many or as few features as they want (or can support, given power constraints). Ideally, pre-built standard authentication and encryption modules will be available from a certification body or third-party software developers [2]. The MDCF should maximize compatibility by offering many security implementations, and should be extensible to ease future integration of evolving technologies. Our modular implementation approach is similar to that of Java or OpenSSL security services [7,8], instantiated by name rather than a function call to a specific method.

Taken together, our modifications to MDCF lay the foundation not only for adding robust authentication and encryption capabilities, but also for easing medical device developer workload by removing the need to write authentication and encryption modules from scratch – pre-defined client-side modules can be used with little or no modification, guaranteeing compatibility as MDCF-side module counterparts have already been implemented.

1.1 Requirements

The purpose of the MDCF device security framework is to serve as an abstraction layer which allows developers to implement different protocols (modules) for device authentication and data confidentiality without having to modify the framework itself. Building such a framework therefore requires some foresight into which MDCF components need to be modified, and how to design the authentication API to be developer-friendly or mostly transparent. Furthermore, we must temporarily maintain backward compatibility (with older devices which do not implement security) as not to break test cases for other ongoing development efforts which use the MDCF.

The MDCF device security framework must hook in to the existing MDCF code base while maintaining backwards compatibility with existing devices. Integration of the device security framework should not require significantly changing the fundamental design/architecture of the MDCF connection state machine or otherwise disturb the overall logical separation of MDCF components – the incorporation of communication security should be mostly or completely transparent to developers working with (or modifying) the MDCF code or message transport layer.

Our target "users" are developers working on new MDCF-compliant devices. They will interact with this framework in two ways: using security providers on devices they create, and/or by creating security providers (**the API should be expressive, powerful, and easy to use**). We will take authentication providers as our example, but data confidentiality (encryption) providers are supported as well. There are multiple authentication providers already implemented and provided for developers. However, we do not prevent developers from building their own authentication modules (**the framework should allow developers to implement arbitrary authentication protocols**), as long as the MDCF can support the protocol (**implementing MDCF authentication modules should not require the alteration of the MDCF**). Finally, we must ensure minimal overhead from the authentication framework (**the only source of overhead should be the authentication modules themselves**, and not the hooks and additional calls to the framework core or messaging layer). In other words, if no authentication happens, no security framework overhead should be visible.

1.2   Authentication Hooks

The MDCF had no implemented security controls when we began, nor was the software written with security in mind. We modified the MDCF to place security "hooks" in several key places in the code to allow for later implementation and deployment of self-contained security modules (similar in spirit to SELinux [9]). The goal was to ensure that these hooks are positioned in a way that allows maintainers to write security modules that are sufficiently "expressive." The MDCF communicates with devices over logical channels, so a natural design choice is to "wrap" the channel in a manner that is transparent to higher-level functions, produce correct output when accessed by an authorized entity, and refuse access to unauthorized users or code.

The resulting modifications to the almost 19,000 lines of the MDCF code base are relatively compact: the security framework (without providers) consists of just over 1,000 lines of code (about 5.56% of the total MDCF). We tested the expressive power of the newly-implemented hooks by first developing a NULL authentication provider, similar to the IPsec NULL encryption method [10], then implementing several other modules, including TLS and DSA. This shows that the security framework is sufficiently flexible to implement almost arbitrary protocols as authentication modules, with an arbitrary number of messages exchanged, all transparent to developers unless they do not use the built-in modules but rather choose to implement their own authentication providers.

1.3   Authentication Providers

Hooks are only part of the solution implementing device authentication in the MDCF. We must also have a component that encapsulates the actual authentication protocol – the authentication provider. All providers implement a common interface so that providers for different protocols can easily be "hooked up." Providers come in pairs – one for the MDCF and another for any device which will support this authentication type, to remove the burden of implementing security-sensitive code from device developers. The provider is responsible for reserving channels to communicate, as well as the actual reception and transmission of messages for its protocol. The device version of the authentication provider, in addition to running the authentication protocol, is also responsible for generating the contents of `authentication` messages sent from a device to the MDCF at the beginning of the connection process. This object identifies the protocol that the device requests to use to authenticate itself. The authentication protocol(s) supported by a device is specified in its metadata, then instantiated by name upon device connection (at runtime). Similarly, the MDCF retrieves its provider by name, based on the protocol specified in a message from the device to the MDCF at device connection time.

1.4 Robustness and Resource Allocation

When implementing authentication protocols, it is important to consider denial of service (DoS) attacks in the form of resource consumption (e.g. SYN flood attack commonly used against web servers [11]). To increase robustness of the MDCF to such attacks, we use the laziest practical resource allocation strategy. For example, one potential first step in device authentication is, upon device connection, to create private channels for this device to communicate with the MDCF. These channels are logical addresses used by the underlying Channel Service, also referred to as the message bus (e.g. OpenJMS, ActiveMQ [12]). Note that this occurs before the device has authenticated successfully, and therefore devices which may never be allowed to communicate with the MDCF can tie up resources either through malice or implementation mistakes. Using only pre-allocated resources (specifically, a pool of pre-allocated authentication providers) until after successful authentication allows us to avoid this problem, so we take special care in placing authentication hooks to minimize resource usage. Malicious devices may keep the pool drained, but honest providers should still be able to eventually connect successfully, with wait times bounded in practice with high probability [13].

2 Background

2.1 ICE

The Integrated Clinical Environment (ICE) is a platform meant to be a ubiquitous standard for medical device interoperability, akin to USB or Wi-Fi in the consumer realm. The goal is to create a functioning system by taking a component-wise approach [2]. In ICE architectures, devices are connected to a component called the Network Controller. This component can be considered the network abstraction: it facilitates communication between devices and applications (automated medical workflows) running on the Supervisor. Figure 1 illustrates the basic architecture of ICE.

The ICE Supervisor hosts apps in isolated environments and guarantees runtime resources like RAM and CPU time. In the ICE architecture, apps are programs that can display patient data as well provide control over devices which support it.

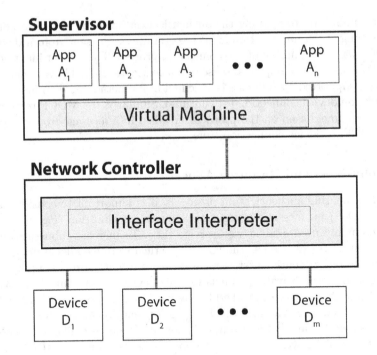

Fig. 1. The primary components of the ICE architecture. External interface, and patient connected to devices, are omitted.

The ICE Network Controller facilitates communication between Supervisor apps and medical devices. All ICE communication takes place through messages sent over virtual channels maintained by the Network Controller (NC). Each channel is specific to a device-app pair. Whenever a new device connects to an ICE system, it is the Network Controller that "discovers" the new device and performs the connection/handshaking and authentication protocols.

2.2 MDCF

The Medical Device Coordination Framework (MDCF) is an open source platform for coordinating and integrating medical devices in order to streamline and automate clinical workflows [5]. The MDCF is intended to be a significant step towards creating a system compliant with the ICE standard. Figure 2 shows the organization of MDCF components with respect to the ICE architecture described in the previous section. They are described in detail below.

Supervisor Components. The App Manager manages the life-cycle of apps; meaning that it starts and stops the execution of apps, provides isolation and service guarantees, monitors and resolves (or notifies clinicians of) "clinically important" (e.g. medically adverse) interactions or architectural interactions (e.g. two apps trying to get exclusive control of one device).

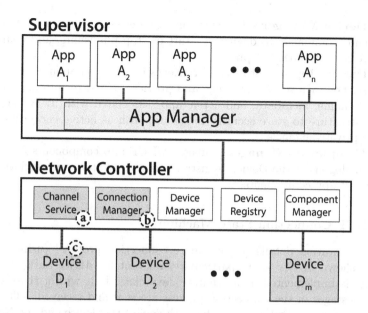

Fig. 2. MDCF components grouped by their logical ICE architecture role and showing primary hook locations (circles a,b,c).

The Clinician Service provides an interface for selecting, instantiating, and configuring Supervisor apps for use with a clinician console GUI. New apps can be started and running ones can be configured. Appropriate user authentication/login will be required.

The Administration Service provides controls for managing and installing Supervisor apps and components. Appropriate user authentication/login will be required. This service should not need to reconfigure running applications, and should be prevented from doing so by the App Manager.

Network Controller Components. The Channel Service provides interfaces between middleware platforms and the rest of the MDCF. It contains interfaces for the messaging server (e.g. OpenJMS, ActiveMQ [12]), message senders, message receivers and message listeners. It is partially responsible for inter-app and inter-device data isolation and performance guarantees. It houses the code for all authentication providers, as well as all interfaces and factories related to authentication providers (Fig. 2(a)).

The Connection Manager manages connections with devices and the creation and destruction of channels through direct interaction with the message provider. The Connection Manager is directly involved with device authentication. It also contains the main hooks for the Network Controller authentication providers (Fig. 2(b)).

The Device Manager sets the status of a device as connected or disconnected, sends commands to devices to start or stop publishing, and configures devices for use with specific apps.

The Device Registry stores and retrieves information about devices from a database. For each device, it stores and provides access to information such as its type, name, metadata, and active apps associated with it. We augment this data structure to store security metadata, such as active encryption keys for device private channels.

The Component Manager manages MDCF app components and works in a way analogous to the Device Registry. It is used to store and retrieve information about app components.

2.3   MDCF Connection State Machine

The implementation details of the device connection protocol (using a state machine), shown in Fig. 3, are particularly relevant for device authentication. Each state is implemented as a separate Java class. It is within these classes that the messages in the connection process are sent and received. Effectively, two connection state machines exist for each device; the device and the Network Controller each maintain their own separate views of this state machine. These different views of the connection state machines are utilized to ensure that all of the steps in connection process are executed in the appropriate order. (In the text, **we refer to the Network Controller view** of the state machine, unless stated otherwise.) Each state machine is associated with a single object that can be used to access or modify the current state. These classes are also used to store any information that needs to be accessed by more than one state. The states most relevant to device authentication are:

DISCONNECTED: The initial state. The device sends the AUTH message during the DISCONNECTED state. Upon reception of the AUTH message, the Network Controller initializes its view of the connection state machine and moves into the AUTHENTICATING state.

AUTHENTICATING: Upon receipt of the AUTH message, the Network Controller allocates and connects to private channels for the device and sends the channel information to the device in an AUTH_ACCEPTED message. The device connects to the channels, after this point the rest of the messages used for connection are sent across these private channels. Note that "private" is used here not to denote confidentiality, but rather than these channels are logically dedicated to communication with a specific device (as opposed to the public "atrium" channel).

AUTHENTICATED: The device has been successfully authenticated. It sends an INTERFACE message to test the private channels before progressing into the ASSOCIATING state. (The INTERFACE message is a confirmation that the private channels set up at the end of the AUTHENTICATING state are working. The content of the message is a fixed string.) Although we routinely

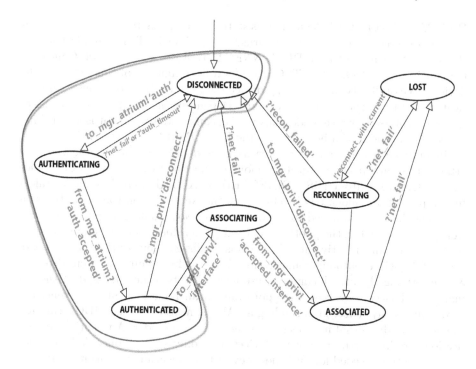

Fig. 3. MDCF Connection State machine, with the outline denoting portions relevant to connection-time authentication.

refer to the device authenticating to the Network Controller, it is trivial to extend the protocol to support mutual authentication.

ASSOCIATING: Upon receipt of the INTERFACE message, the Network Controller creates heartbeat and acknowledgment channels. The device periodically publishes heartbeat messages on this channel, enabling the Network Controller to detect an unexpected device disconnection (if too many heartbeat messages are missing). The Network Controller communicates these private heartbeat channels to the device and then transitions to the ASSOCIATED state.

ASSOCIATED: The device is fully connected in this state. The device will remain in this state unless it ceases to be connected and transitions to either the LOST or DISCONNECTED state.

LOST: When too many device heartbeats have been lost, the Network Controller places the device in the LOST state. It must then attempt to reconnect, transitioning into the RECONNECTING state. (If the device state machine is not in the LOST state, and it successfully communicated with the Network Controller, it will be explicitly told to reconnect.)

RECONNECTING: A device in this state is attempting to reconnect. If reconnection is successful, the device it returns to the ASSOCIATED state. Otherwise, the device transitions to the DISCONNECTED state. The Network Controller remains in the RECONNECTING state for a fixed amount of time, or until the device successfully reconnects. Only devices which have been previously authenticated may be in the reconnecting state. Depending on the specific authentication protocol used, device credentials may become "stale" while it is attempting to reconnect, and it will be moved to the DISCONNECTED state.

In practice, to minimize resource usage and protect against resource DoS attacks, the state machine object used for a connection by the Network Controller (in the transition from DISCONNECTED to AUTHENTICATING) is taken from a pool of pre-allocated objects. When the Network Controller "destroys" a state machine, it is returned to the object pool. Note that this prevents devices from connecting when the pool is exhausted (either due to a large number of connected devices or an active attack). This is by design: devices that authenticate successfully will eventually connect, and devices which cannot authenticate but are performing the attack cannot cause more objects to be allocated. Although malicious devices may keep the pool drained, an honest client will eventually (probabilistically) succeed in sending an AUTH message to the MDCF through the flood of adversarial messages, thus reserving a provider. Authenticated connections are long-term, so honest devices need only succeed once. When under attack, the time needed for an honest device to connect may be arbitrarily long, but in practice would be bounded with high probability [13].

3 Security Design

3.1 Device Authentication Hooks

The MDCF connection state machine, before the introduction of authentication, automatically transitioned from the AUTHENTICATING state to the AUTHENTICATED state (without implementing authentication). To make authentication as seamless as possible for MDCF developers, hooks were placed such that all authentication protocols are executed while in the AUTHENTICATING state. Although authentication protocols themselves may involve multiple rounds of message exchange, this is hidden and encapsulated by the AUTHENTICATING state. The net result is that a full authentication protocol can be implemented without requiring any changes to the remainder of the system, provided any communication channel between the device and Network Controller have already been set up.

To make this possible, hooks are placed so that the protocol is executed after the AUTH message is exchanged but before the AUTH_ACCEPTED message is sent. These messages are sent and received within the DISCONNECTED and AUTHENTICATING states. Therefore, the primary location for the hooks is within the connection state machine. Our API does not enforce any restrictions on either the number of rounds or the content of messages exchanged by authentication providers. Thus the framework satisfies the requirement that developers are allowed to implement arbitrary authentication protocols. Because it is possible to implement arbitrary authentication protocols, developers may create providers which facilitate server authentication in addition to the standard client (device) authentication. An authentication provider factory is initialized at runtime, and a provider pool (with at least one provider) is ready when a device calls the provider at connection time. The provider is fetched by name (requested by the connecting device) from the pool and executed from within the DISCONNECTED and AUTHENTICATING states. The AUTH message contains an `authentication` object that stores two pieces of information: a value specifying the authentication protocol requested by the device, and the device's public key.

In addition to the hooks described above, an additional message must be sent from the Network Controller to the device across the atrium channel (used by all devices upon initial connection). This message, called the AUTH_PROTOCOL message, was required as part of this implementation. It contains information about the channels that will be used by the authentication provider to execute an authentication protocol and may also include other information such as the public key of the Network Controller. The authentication providers have access to two channels with which they can communicate with each other. The NULL authentication providers currently make use of the public atrium channels, `from_mgr_atrium` and `to_mgr_atrium`. It should be noted that these channels were used out of convenience for this initial implementation, but they are ill suited for this purpose because every message sent on `from_mgr_atrium` is effectively broadcast to all other devices leading to unnecessary communication overhead. Future authentication providers will use private channels instead. Authentication providers execute their protocol when their respective `runAuthProtocol()` methods are called. (Note that this is not a security risk, as all messages between the MDCF and the device would be end-to-end encrypted and authenticated in a production system.) The connection state machines wait for these methods to return boolean values to indicate either a successful or failed authentication attempt. If the authentication fails then the device is disconnected, otherwise, the device resumes the connection process.

The location of the authentication hooks also allows us to ensure that authentication can not be bypassed (unless disabled totally by a system administrator). The only way that a device can connect to the MDCF is by progressing through the correct sequence of states in the connection state machine. The sequence of states can be seen in Fig. 3. A device begins in the DISCONNECTED state. From there, it may only transition to the AUTHENTICATING state. A device in the AUTHENTICATING state must enter the DISCONNECTED state if authentication fails, or AUTHENTICATED if it succeeds. Each device must go through the AUTHENTICATING state in order to connect. The authentication hooks are placed such that an authentication provider must execute before a device can transition from AUTHENTICATING to AUTHENTICATED, therefore authentication may not be bypassed.

3.2   Message Confidentiality and Authenticity Hooks

In addition to the authentication hooks, we have added hooks for channel security providers. These providers allow us to gain confidentiality through message encryption, and enforce and verify the integrity and authenticity of messages using digital signatures or message authentication codes. (Although the channel security providers are an essential part of the overall MDCF security architecture, we primarily focus on evaluating authentication providers in this work.)

To gain these additional security properties, we position hooks within the channel service so that every message sent or received by a device or app must pass through a channel security provider. Each channel security provider is able to apply arbitrary transformations on a message, so we can transparently encrypt, decrypt, and authenticate messages. During the initialization of a message sender or receiver, it is bound to a channel security provider, ensuring that security-related transformations on messages may not be bypassed. Channel security providers come in pairs – one for sending a message and another for receiving a message. The application of these providers is on a channel-by-channel basis, making it possible to extend this feature to provide fine-grained control over how confidentiality, integrity, and authenticity are enforced for each channel. We envision that a device's long term keys, obtained during device authentication, will be stored within the Device Registry. These long term keys might then be used in some way to derive short term keys for encryption and message authenticity/integrity. To date, we have implemented a NULL channel security provider, which performs no operations on a message, and another one which uses Java's built in TLS provider, which is passed to the channel security providers from the TLS authentication provider.

3.3   NULL Authentication Provider

To check the overhead of our design and the expressiveness of the hooks, we implemented a NULL authentication provider, which authenticates successfully if it receives a message "PONG" in response to its challenge "PING." The execution of the provider is mapped out in Fig. 4 and described below.

1. The MDCF and device initialize. The MDCF initializes providers and populates its provider pool.
2. The device fetches any[1] supported authentication method from the device-side authentication provider object, then composes and sends an AUTH message to the Network Controller (NC) with the name of the authentication algorithm.

---

[1] Multiple methods may be supported both by the device and the MDCF, but currently negotiation is not implemented.

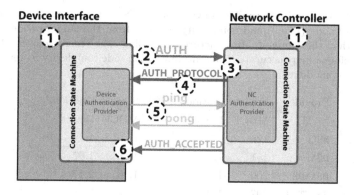

Fig. 4. Illustration of the authentication process using the NULL provider.

3. Upon reception of the AUTH message, the NC creates its own view of the connection state machine for this device. It then fetches the appropriate pre-initialized authentication provider from the provider pool, and passes the contents of the AUTH message to this provider.
4. The NC-side authentication provider obtains channels to be used for executing the authentication protocol with the device. It then sends an AUTH_PROTOCOL message to the device that specifies which channels should be used by the authentication protocol only (the device is assigned new channels after it successfully authenticates).
5. The protocol is executed, for the NULL authentication provider, which simply consists of an exchange of the strings "PING" and "PONG" between the device and NC.
6. Upon successful competition of the protocol, the NC creates new private channels for the device, sending the handles of those channels to the device in an AUTH_ACCEPTED message.

In addition to our NULL provider, we implemented three "non-trivial" providers for evaluation purposes: SSL/TLS, DSA, and DSA+DH. This exercise allowed us to confirm that we meet two of our stated requirements. We found that the API is sufficiently expressive, powerful, and easy to use. Also, as we explain later in this section, we found the only source of overhead comes from the authentication modules themselves. Compared to developing and implementing the framework, creating a provider is relatively simple, e.g. our SSL/TLS provider is only 207 lines of Java code. It is based on Oracle's java.net.ssl implementation, running TLS 1.2 and using the TLS_DHE_DSS_WITH_AES_128_CBC_SHA cipher suite. This implementation can be trivially expanded to support mutual authentication with only a few additional lines of code (SSL/TLS provides this as standard functionality). Code length metrics for all providers are in Table 1. The other two authentication providers (DSA and DSA+DH) use a simple challenge-response protocol in which a message from the device to the Network Controller includes a DSA signature from the device. Upon receiving this message, the Network Controller verifies the signature and then sends a signed response message

Table 1. Authentication provider (device- and MDCF-side), complexity measured using lines of code (LOC), and complexity increase from the NULL provider. NULL is little more than the common infrastructure/scaffolding. The "Increase over NULL" column is therefore a more accurate representation of the code complexity increase of new authentication modules.

Provider	Implementation (LOC)		Increase over NULL	
	MDCF	Device	MDCF	Device
NULL	128	72	1	1
DSA	151	120	1.18	1.67
DSA+DH	200	178	1.56	2.47
SSL/TLS	207	171	1.62	2.38

to the device. Once the device verifies this response, the authentication protocol terminates – note that this is a mutual authentication protocol.

4   Evaluation

In order to confirm that we meet the requirement of overhead in the authentication system stemming only from the authentication modules themselves, we ran performance tests of our modified MDCF implementation on a server with dual hex-core Intel Xeon X5670 64-bit CPUs at roughly 2.93 GHz, with 12 MB cache and 24 GB system RAM, running Linux 3.8.13 and Sun's Java virtual machine version 1.7.0_21. The resulting performance is shown in Fig. 5. Due to the limitations of Java and the current MDCF architecture on our testbed, we could only reliably test 340 or fewer concurrent devices. In an attempt to tax the resources of the MDCF and our authentication providers, the initial sharp spike in resource usage is due to all test devices attempting to connect simultaneously. Each device begins sending physiological data (SpO2 and pulse rate) following a successful join.

Figures 5(a) and (c) show the resource usage of MDCF using unauthenticated connections. The Y axis are constrained for readability. The highest observed CPU utilization within the startup "spike" was 16% (DSA). Figures 5(b) and (d) show the resources used after including framework hooks only (control) and when using various authentication providers. The highest CPU utilization within the startup spike was 19.75% (TLS), with DSA and DSA+DH reaching 17.4% and 16.7%, respectively. Each line represents an average of 11 instances of tests using identical configurations with 340 devices (device-side performance not shown for readability). The standard error is negligible (the difference between lines is statistically significant), and error bars have been omitted for clarity. The control is a version of MDCF without any authentication code at all – the authentication code was not disabled, but rather removed entirely to avoid unexpected interactions.

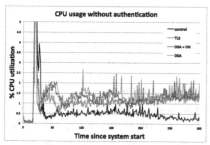

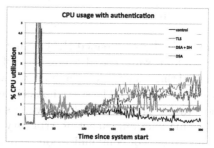

(a) MDCF processor usage with all devices permitted

(b) MDCF processor usage with only authenticated devices permitted

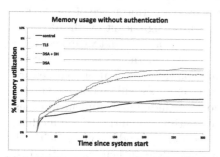

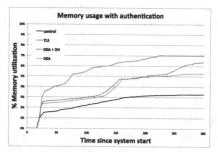

(c) MDCF memory usage with all devices permitted

(d) MDCF memory usage with only authenticated devices permitted

Fig. 5. MDCF resource usage with 340 virtual devices running on a different host.

The entire authentication framework consumes negligible resources – indistinguishable from control, satisfying our requirement. Authentication modules in Figs. 5(a) and (c) show a modest but fixed resource cost. They are included in the running code, and a fixed number are initialized to populate the provider pool, but are inactive – devices do not include authentication code and therefore never request to authenticate (backward compatibility mode). Running authentication modules impose an increase in resource usage dependent on the specific protocol being used (resource usage is protocol-dependent).

The network overhead in terms of latency and traffic volume is highly dependent on the individual protocol being used, and can be tuned (by selecting the appropriate protocol) depending on requirements. Authentication imposes a one-time latency increase due to the larger number of network round trips required at connection time, but the observable slowdown is negligible, and only occurs once – upon initial device connection. We found that only the TLS provider caused an increase in bandwidth usage, but to such a small extent as not to interfere with normal operation.

5 Conclusion

In this work we extended the existing MDCF high-assurance medical coordination middleware to add a flexible and modular authentication framework, and showed that, in practice, the framework scaffolding itself adds negligible overhead at execution time. The set of hooks introduced into the MDCF, while minimal, is nonetheless sufficiently expressive to support the design and integration of arbitrary modules implementing arbitrary authentication protocols using arbitrarily many rounds of communication before passing control back to the body of the MDCF. Moreover, the code is fully concurrent – devices do not have to wait "in line" to authenticate, but are handled at the same time. Authentication requests can be processed simultaneously, limited only by the performance of the MDCF itself, as authentication scaffolding did not result in significant overhead.

While we do not implement the authentication protocols that we expect to be used in practice (ours are somewhat simplified), we nonetheless observe that the framework itself does not impose undue burden on the coordination middleware, and therefore the performance of future security modules will be bounded by the efficiency of those protocols themselves and their individual implementations, not the cost of dynamic dispatch and call-at-runtime semantics of the modular security framework. Auto-generation of device module code from MDCF-side code, as well as implementing and measuring individual authentication protocol performance on the MDCF and device sides is left up to future work. Further, our current providers rely on pre-shared certificates, but in practice this may not be the case – a "true" Plug-n-Play device, connecting for the first time, will have to transmit its certificate, leading to greater network overhead. Developing and evaluating full certificate trust chain verification is likewise future work.

Acknowledgments. The authors would like to thank Daniel Andresen for his input and help in testing the prototype. The computing for this project was performed on the Beocat Research Cluster at Kansas State University, which is funded in part by NSF grants CNS 1006860, EPS 1006860, and EPS 0919443. This research was supported in part by the NIH grant 1U01EB012470-01 and NSF awards CNS 1126709, CNS 1224007, and CNS 1253930.

References

1. Hatcliff, J., Vasserman, E., Weininger, S., Goldman, J.: An overview of regulatory and trust issues for the integrated clinical environment. In: Joint Workshop On High Confidence Medical Devices, Software, and Systems and Medical Device Plug-and-Play Interoperability (HCMDSS/MD PnP) (2011)
2. Hatcliff, J., King, A., Lee, I., MacDonald, A., Fernando, A., Robkin, M., Vasserman, E.Y., Weininger, S., Goldman, J.M.: Rationale and architecture principles for medical application platforms. In: International Conference on Cyber-Physical Systems (ICCPS) (2012)
3. Conmy, P., Nicholson, M., McDermid, J.: Safety assurance contracts for integrated modular avionics. In: Australian Workshop on Safety Critical Systems and Software (SCS), vol. 33 (2003)

4. ASTM Committee F-29, Anaesthetic and Respiratory Equipment, Subcommittee 21, Devices in the integrated clinical environment: Medical devices and medical systems – essential safety requirements for equipment comprising the patient-centric integrated clinical environment (ICE) (2009)

5. King, A., Procter, S., Andresen, D., Hatcliff, J., Warren, S., Spees, W., Jetley, R., Jones, P., Weininger, S.: An open test bed for medical device integration and coordination. In: International Conference on Software Engineering (ICSE) (2009)

6. Arney, D., Weininger, S., Whitehead, S.F., Goldman, J.M.: Supporting medical device adverse event analysis in an interoperable clinical environment: design of a data logging and playback system. In: International Conference on Biomedical Ontology (ICBO) (2011)

7. Gong, L., Ellison, G.: Inside Java(TM) 2 Platform Security: Architecture, API Design, and Implementation, 2nd edn. Pearson Education, Upper Saddle River (2003)

8. OpenSSL: OpenSSL: Documents, ssl(3) (2012). https://www.openssl.org/docs/ssl/ssl.html

9. McCarty, B.: SELinux: NSA's Open Source Security Enhanced Linux. O'Reilly, Sebastopol (2005)

10. Glenn, R., Kent, S.: The NULL encryption algorithm and its use with IPsec (1998)

11. Schuba, C.L., Krsul, I.V., Kuhn, M.G., Spafford, E.H., Sundaram, A., Zamboni, D.: Analysis of a denial of service attack on TCP. In: IEEE Symposium on Security and Privacy (1997)

12. Snyder, B., Bosanac, D., Davies, R.: ActiveMQ in Action. Manning Publications, Manning Pubs Co Series, Manning (2011)

13. Millen, J.K.: A resource allocation model for denial of service. In: IEEE Symposium on Security and Privacy (1992)

Towards an AADL-Based Definition of App Architecture for Medical Application Platforms

Sam Procter[⊠], John Hatcliff, and Robby

Kansas State University, Manhattan, KS, USA
{samprocter,hatcliff,robby}@ksu.edu

Abstract. There is a growing trend of developing software applications that integrate and coordinate the actions of medical devices. Unfortunately, these applications are being built in an ad-hoc manner without proper regard for established distributed systems engineering techniques. We present a tool prototype based on the OSATE2 distribution of the Eclipse IDE that targets the development of Medical Application Platform (MAP) apps. Our toolset provides an editing environment and translator for app architectures, i.e., their components and connections. The toolset generates interface definitions and glue code for the underlying MAP middleware, and it supports development of the business logic which the developer must write to complete the application within the same Eclipse-based environment. We also present a clinical scenario as a motivating example, trace its development through the toolset, and evaluate our work based on the experience.

Keywords: Integrated medical systems · Medical application platforms · Software architecture · AADL

1 Introduction

Medical devices, which have traditionally been built and certified in a stand-alone fashion, are beginning to be integrated with one another in various ways: information from one device is forwarded to another for display, information from multiple devices is combined to get a more accurate representation of a patient's health, or a device may even monitor or interrupt routine treatments (e.g., administration of an analgesic) via "closed-loop" execution. The architecture of these systems has begun to attract the attention of regulatory and certification agencies; the FDA now recognizes ASTM's F2761 standard [4], which lays out a functional architecture for an integrated clinical environment (ICE). Implementation of these systems is increasingly realized on some sort of real-time middleware, leading to important realizations about commonalities and differences between them and other, more traditional, distributed systems.

This work is supported in part by the US National Science Foundation (NSF) (#1239543), the NSF US Food and Drug Administration Scholar-in-Residence Program (#1355778) and the National Institutes of Health / NIBIB Quantum Program.

© Springer International Publishing AG 2017
M. Huhn and L. Williams (Eds.): FHIES 2014/SEHC 2014, LNCS 9062, pp. 26–43, 2017.
DOI: 10.1007/978-3-319-63194-3_3

Consider the following scenario which has been identified and studied in the literature that we will use as a motivating example throughout this work [15]:

> After an uneventful hysterectomy, a patient was given a patient-controlled analgesia (PCA) pump to deliver morphine. However, too much of the drug was administered even after her vital signs had become depressed and she ultimately died [5]. The pump could have been disabled and the patient's life saved had a simple monitoring algorithm had access to her physiological monitors and been capable of disabling her PCA pump.

The term medical application platform (MAP) was introduced in [11], where it was defined as a "safety- and security-critical real-time computing platform for: (a) integrating heterogeneous devices, medical IT systems, and information displays via a communication infrastructure, and (b) hosting application programs (i.e. apps) that provide medical utility via the ability to both acquire information from and update/control integrated devices, IT systems, and displays." Similar to [11], we focus on MAPs in a clinical context, though we envision their potential use in "portable, home-based, mobile or distributed [systems]."

Although work has been done on application requirements [19] and the architecture of MAPs [11,17], little attention has been paid to the architectures of medical applications (apps) that run on a MAP. These MAP apps are essentially new medical devices that are: (a) specified by an application developer, (b) instantiated at the point of care, and (c) coordinated by the MAP itself. Most of the previously built applications on these prototype platforms were designed in an ad-hoc manner with the goal of demonstrating certain functionality concepts.

What is needed is to move from this ad-hoc approach to something that can enable systematic engineering and reuse. Such an approach would enable true component-based development, which would utilize network-aware devices as services on top of a real-time, publish-subscribe middleware. These devices could be composed by an application at runtime to define the medical system's behavior, though this would require careful reasoning about the architecture of the application.

While this sort of careful reasoning about the architecture of MAP apps (also referred to as *virtual medical devices*) has not been performed before, the architecture of other bus-based, safety-critical systems has been given a great deal of attention. The *Architecture Analysis & Design Language* (AADL) was released in November 2004 by the Society of Automotive Engineers (SAE) as aerospace standard AS5506 [8]. Described as "a modeling language that supports early and repeated analyses of a system's architecture... through an extendable notation, a tool framework, and precisely defined semantics," it enables developers to model the architecture of the hardware and software aspects of a system as well as their integration.[1] That is, not only can processors and processes be modeled, but so can the mapping from the latter to the former. It has found some success in systems development in both the aerospace (e.g., the "integrate then build"

---

[1] Moreover, there are language annexes which enable the specification of a system's behavior in AADL.

approach undertaken in the SAVI effort [10]) and automotive fields, and it has even been applied to the development of traditional medical devices [14,21].

Since MAP app development is in need of more engineering rigor and AADL was developed to provide architectural modeling and analysis for safety-critical systems, it seems natural to evaluate their combined use. Additionally, AADL has an established community and has been hardened by nearly a decade of use (see Sect. 3.2). However, it is not immediately clear whether a technology aimed at the integration of hardware and software in the automotive and aerospace industries will be applicable to the domain of MAP apps. For example, since MAPs do not expose the raw hardware of their platform—rather programming abstractions above it—it is unclear how well certain AADL features will work when only these software abstractions are being modeled, or if they will be necessary at all.

What is needed, then, is: (a) a subset of AADL that is useful when describing the architecture of MAP apps, and (b) a supporting set of tools to facilitate app development. We describe an approach and prototype toolset using a publicly available, open source MAP called the *Medical Device Coordination Framework* (MDCF [2]); while being specific to MDCF, we believe our work generalizes to other rigorously engineered MAPs.

Specifically, the main contributions of this paper are:

1. A proposed subset of the full AADL (selected components and port-based communication) that is useful for describing a MAP app's architecture.
2. A proposal for a set of properties necessary for describing the real-time (RT) and quality-of-service (QoS) properties of MAP apps. This set includes some of AADL's built-in properties, and it also utilizes AADL's property description mechanism to specify new properties.
3. An implementation of a translator that takes as input the relevant properties and app component structure (as identified in 1 and 2) and produces as output an application context for the MDCF. Specifically, the translator produces code that automatically: (a) configures the underlying publish-subscribe middleware of the MDCF, (b) configures the components to work together as described in the architectural model, and (c) enforces the RT and QoS parameters via properties described in (2).
4. A runnable app which demonstrates the expected translator output and implements the previously discussed clinical scenario. The architecture of the app is specified in our proposed subset of AADL and the output is runnable on the MDCF.

The remainder of this paper is organized as follows. Section 2 outlines our overall app development vision. Section 3 provides a background on technologies and problems relevant to this work, chiefly MAPs and AADL. Section 4 gives a walkthrough of the supported language subset and relevant properties. Finally, Sect. 5 concludes and describes future work.

2   Vision

At the center of our long-term MAP app development vision is an *App Development Environment* (ADE) that is built on an industrial grade Integrated Development Environment (IDE) which supports model-driven development of apps. The IDE should provide access to traditional software development tools including editors, compilers, debuggers, and testing infrastructure. The ADE should also have a pluggable architecture so that a variety of components for supporting app analysis, verification, and artifact construction can be easily added to the environment. Additionally, the envisioned ADE should enable compilation and packaging of an app so that it can be directly deployed and executed on a MAP such as the MDCF.

In addition to supporting traditional development, an important aspect of our vision is that the ADE should support preparation of a variety of artifacts required in third-party certification and regulatory approval of the app. For example, the ADE should support the construction of requirements documents with capabilities that would enable requirements to be traced to both individual features and formal specifications in the app model and implementation. The ADE should support preparation of hazard and risk analysis artifacts (which should also be traceable to models/code). We envision a variety of forms of verification such as (a) app-to-device interface compatibility checking, (b) component implementation to component contract conformance verification, (c) model checking of real-time aspects of concurrent interactions, (d) error and hazard modeling using AADL's EMV2 annex [18], and (e) proof environments that support full-functional correctness proofs for an app. The ADE should also support construction of rigorous styles of argumentation, such as assurance cases (again, with traceability links to other artifacts).

Additionally, the envisioned ADE would aid in preparation of third-party certification and regulatory submission documents (e.g., the FDA 510(k)), as well as the packaging of artifacts into digitally-signed archives that could be shipped to relevant entities. These organizations would be able to use the same framework to browse the submitted artifacts and re-run testing and verification tools. The work presented in this paper represents the first step towards achieving this vision.

3   Background

Our work on this topic was guided by our experiences with the state of medical application platforms (primarily the MDCF), interest in AADL, previous work with safety-critical software engineering and the associated regulatory oversight, and requirements engineering for MAP apps [19].

3.1   Medical Application Platforms

The concept of MAPs predates the term; one notable publication is the ASTM standard F2761, which introduces one possible MAP architecture, referred to as the *Integrated Clinical Environment* (ICE) [4]. A logical view of an app running

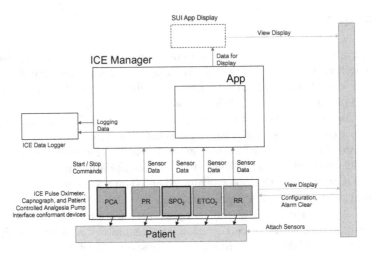

Fig. 1. The PCA Interlock App's information flows. The devices used in the app excerpt discussed in this section have bolded borders.

on the ICE architecture is given in Fig. 1. The ICE manager, which consists of a supervisor and network controller, provides a configurable execution context upon which apps can run and is supported by a real-time middleware that can guarantee various timing and QoS properties. Devices connected to an ICE system can be used (or controlled) by the apps running on the manager, and various services (e.g., logging and display functionality) are provided transparently to the app. There are a number of implementations of the ICE architecture including the MDCF [16] as well as commercial offerings like Dräger's BICEPS [23].

MAP Applications: MAP applications, as distributed systems, are built using the traditional "components and connections" style of systems engineering. Any development environment for apps, then, should have a number of *core features* that are important to component-based development:

- *Support for well-defined interfaces:* The components of distributed systems should be self-contained, with the exception of the inputs and outputs they expose over well-defined interfaces. This enables a library of commonly used components to be made available to the developer.
- *Support for common patterns of communication:* Not only are the components of such a system often reusable, but so are the styles of communication between the components. Adhering to common patterns will also result in a more straightforward software verification process.
- *Support for real-time and quality-of-service configuration:* In a real-time, safety-critical distributed system, correctness requires not only the right information, but also getting it at the right time. Safety arguments can be difficult to make without the ability to set expected timings in an app's configuration

(e.g., a task's worst-case execution time) and have a guarantee of the enforcement of those timings from the underlying middleware.

The translator and example artifact portions of this work target the MDCF because it supports a rigorous notion of component specification. Since the MIDdleware Assurance Substrate (MIDAS) [3] is one of the middleware frameworks supported by the MDCF, our translator supports setting a range of timing properties attached to both connections (e.g., a port's latency) and components (e.g., a task's worst-case execution time). As previously noted, though, the work described here is not deeply tied to the MDCF but could be targeted to any MAP implementation that supports similarly rigorous notions of component definition, configuration, and communication.

We believe the *core concepts* common to specifications of app architectures are:

- *Layout:* A high-level schema that defines how various components connect to one another and collectively form the app.
- *Medical Device:* Individual medical devices which will either be controlled by software components, or produce physiological information that will be consumed by software components.
- *Software Component:* Software pieces that typically (though not exclusively) consume physiological information and produce clinically meaningful output (e.g., information for a display, smart alarms, or commands to medical devices).
- *Channel:* Routes through a network over which components (i.e., both medical devices and software) can communicate.

Taken together, the core features and concepts enable reusability by ensuring that components communicate over interfaces in common, pattern-based ways with strict timing constraints. A component is capable of interoperating in any other system where it "fits." That is, its interface exposes the required ports, utilizes the same communication patterns, and has compatible timing requirements.

3.2   Architecture Analysis and Design Language

SAE's AADL is a standardized, model-based engineering language that was developed for safety-critical system engineering. Therefore, it has a number of features that make it particularly well suited to our needs:

- *Hierarchical refinement:* AADL supports the notion of first defining an element and then further refining it into a decomposition of several subcomponents. This will not only keep the modelling elements more clean and readable, but will also allow app creators to work in a top-down style of development. They will be able to first think about what components make up the system and how those components might be linked together, then define those components, and finally reason about how those individual components would themselves be comprised.

Table 1. AADL syntax elements in our subset and their MAP app mappings

AADL construct	MAP concept	Mapping explanation
Components		
System	Layout	This equivalence is not a large stretch, as systems "[represent] a composite that can include... components" [7]
Device	Device	This is essentially a direct equivalence
Process	Software Component	AADL processes "[represent] a protected address space that [prevents] other components from accessing anything inside." [7] Our language uses processes to group related tasks into a single component
Thread	Task	Tasks represent some unit of work to be done either periodically or upon arrival of a message on a designated port. Tasks are local to their containing process, allowing them to share state, but stopping them from directly manipulating tasks or state outside their enclosing process
Connections		
System	Channel	Channels enable communication between components, using a messaging service
Process	Task Trigger	Message arrival on an `event` or `event data` port triggers an associated task, while `data` ports simply update a predictably-named field
Process impl.	Task-Port Comm.	A port connection from a process to a thread translates to a task's use of data arriving via that port

- *Distinction between types and implementations:* AADL allows a developer to first define a component and then give it one or more implementations, similar to the object-oriented programming practice of first defining an interface and then creating one or more implementations of that interface. This keeps app models cleaner and enables code reuse.
- *Extensible property system:* AADL allows developers to create properties, specify their type, and restrict which constructs they can be attached to. We have used this feature to, for example, associate various physiological parameters with their IEEE 11073 nomenclature "tag" [12].
- *Textual and graphical representations:* AADL has a defined textual and graphical syntax, and there is tool support for converting between the two representations.
- *Strong tool support:* AADL is supported by a wide range of both open source (e.g., OSATE2 [22]) and commercial (e.g., STOOD [6]) tools. We have used OSATE2 as the basis for our toolset, and have found a number of its features quite useful (e.g., element name auto-completion, type-checking, etc.).

In general, AADL models are composed of components and their connections. AADL includes a number of software modeling entities (e.g., thread, process, data, etc.), hardware entities (e.g., processor, memory, device, etc.), and composite entities (e.g., system and abstract). AADL also includes connections between components of various types such as ports, data accesses, bus accesses, etc. Of these, our language and translator use only a small subset: the system, device, process and thread entities, and port communication. Elements outside of this subset are either not needed for app construction (e.g., the flows entity) or may be added later (e.g., the subprogram entity). The mapping from these constructs to the MAP constructs identified in Sect. 3.1 is listed in Table 1; a full explanation of how our subset is used to define an app is given in the next section.

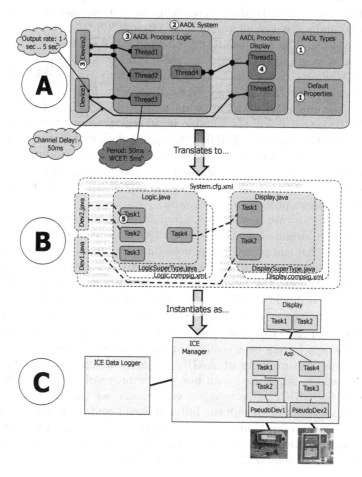

Fig. 2. (A) The AADL platform artifacts used by the code generation process, (B) the generated app configuration and executable files, and (C) the fully configured and executing platform.

4   Language Walkthrough

In this section, we describe the process of creating a MAP app with our prototype toolset using the motivating example of the PCA Interlock app initially described in Sect. 1. This app consumes various physiological parameters to determine the health of the patient and disables the flow of an analgesic when there are indications of respiratory failure [20]. A high-level, ICE-configuration/logical view of the app is shown in Fig. 1. The diagram shows that in addition to the PCA pump, there are four sensors: (i) a blood-oxygen saturation (SpO_2) sensor, (ii) a pulse rate sensor, (iii) a respiratory rate sensor, and (iv) an end-tidal carbon dioxide ($ETCO_2$) sensor. In this application, the sensors may be on the same device: SpO_2 and pulse rate information are often produced by a pulse oximeter (e.g., the Ivy 450C [13]), and respiratory rate and $ETCO_2$ information can come from, e.g., a capnography machine (e.g., the Capnostream 20 [1]).

The PCA pump consumes information from the app (e.g., enable and disable commands) while the others produce information in the form of sensor data that are used by the app's logic. An important part of the app (and the underlying MAP/MDCF) is that it will use suitable physiological parameters regardless of their source; that is, instead of building the app to work with a specific device or set of devices, it is built to work with a generic source of the required physiological parameters. We hope to present the process for deriving/documenting the requirements (e.g., the topic of [19]) that were used to create this diagram/drive the app development process in future work.

Figure 2 gives an overview of the app architecture development, code generation, and app instantiation process. Part (A) of the figure shows the various AADL artifacts that compose the app; note that they are labeled with the number of the subsection they are discussed in. Part (B) shows the execution and configuration artifacts that result from code generation. It also highlights the large number of components (signified by dashed lines) that are fully automatically generated. Part (C) shows the app's instantiation on a running MAP, first sketched in Fig. 1, with both the computation hosting and communication aspects of the app having been realized in the ICE architecture.

We now present excerpts of AADL models that specify the application architecture which, when used with our translator, results in application code runnable on the MDCF. Due to space constraints, we only show one physiological parameter, SpO_2, though the full app would contain all four parameters (i.e., SpO_2, pulse rate, respiratory rate, and $ETCO_2$). In the next subsection, we discuss AADL types and default properties, followed by a top-down walkthrough of the hierarchy of components used by our toolset.

4.1   Preliminary Tasks: Types and Default Properties

Before we can describe a MAP app's architecture, we must briefly examine AADL's type and property definition mechanisms (marked by a (1) in Fig. 2) and how they are used to specify various parameters in our app.

```
 1  package PCA_Interlock_Types
 2  public
 3  with Data_Model, IEEE11073_Nomenclature;
 4    data SpO2
 5    properties
 6      Data_Model::Data_Representation => Integer;
 7      IEEE11073_Nomenclature::OID => IEEE11073_Nomenclature::MDC_PULS_OXIM_SAT_O2;
 8      Data_Model::Integer_Range => 0 .. 100;
 9    end SpO2;
10  end PCA_Interlock_Types;
```

(a) The SpO$_2$ datatype used in the app excerpt

```
 1  property set PCA_Interlock_Properties is
 2    with PCA_Interlock;
 3    Default_Thread_Time : constant Time => 50 ms;
 4    Default_Output_Rate : Time_Range => 100 ms .. 300 ms applies to (port);
 5    Default_Thread_Dispatch : Supported_Dispatch_Protocols => Sporadic applies to (
          thread);
 6    Default_Thread_Period : Time => PCA_Interlock_Properties::Default_Thread_Time
          applies to (thread);
 7    Default_Thread_Deadline : Time => PCA_Interlock_Properties::Default_Thread_Time
          applies to (thread);
 8    Default_Thread_WCET : Time => 5 ms applies to (thread);
 9    Default_Channel_Delay : Time => 100 ms applies to ({PCA_Interlock} ** port
          connection);
10  end PCA_Interlock_Properties;
```

(b) The default properties used in the app excerpt

Fig. 3. Data types and default properties used in the app excerpt

Data Types: The data type for the SpO$_2$ parameter is shown in Fig. 3a. AADL's property description mechanism is easily extensible, allowing us to specify customer-specific metadata. In this example, we have leveraged this capability to attach an IEEE 11073 nomenclature "tag" with our SpO$_2$ parameter [12]. Note that these datatypes could either be generated from or mapped down to a more standard interface definition language (e.g., CORBA IDL [24]).

Default Property Values: While it is useful to be able to attach properties to individual AADL constructs (e.g., ports, connections, threads, etc.), sometimes a large number of constructs take the same values for certain properties. In this case, it is useful to set app-wide defaults, as shown in Fig. 3b. Unless overridden, these properties will apply to every applicable element. A full listing of default and override property names and types is shown in Table 2.

4.2 The AADL System

The top level of the app architecture is described by an AADL system, marked by a ② in Fig. 2, and shown textually in Fig. 4. In our subset of AADL, systems have no external features (lines 4–5), though the system implementation lists their internals (lines 7–20). An AADL system implementation consists of a declaration of sub-components (e.g., devices and processes), the connections between them, and optionally a description of the paths (flows) data take through the system. Note that we show only excerpts; other interactions include alarm/alert communication

Table 2. AADL property names, types, examples, and explanations

Default Name	Type	Example	Explanation
Override Name			
Thread Properties			
Default_Thread_Period	Time	50 ms	Periodic tasks will be dispatched to run once per period
Timing_Properties::Period			
Default_Thread_Deadline	Time	50 ms	A task will be scheduled such that it has time to complete before its deadline
Timing_Properties::Deadline			
Default_Thread_WCET	Time	50 ms	A task's worst case execution time is the most time it will take to complete after dispatch
Timing_Properties::Compute_Execution_Time			
Default_Thread_Dispatch	Sporadic or Periodic	Periodic	Periodic tasks are dispatched once per period, sporadic upon message arrival
Thread_Properties::Dispatch_Protocol			
Port Properties			
Default_Output_Rate	Time Range	100 ms .. 300 ms	Ports must specify the most and least frequently that they will broadcast a message
MAP_Properties::Output_Rate			
Port Connection Properties			
Default_Channel_Delay	Time	100 ms	Specifies the maximum time that the message can spend on the network
MAP_Properties::Channel_Delay			
Process Properties			
N/A	Logic or Display	Display	Processes are either for logic or display components
MAP_Properties::Component_Type			

and parameter setting. Flows (line 22 of Fig. 4, line 10 of Fig. 5, and line 8 of Fig. 6) allow a developer to trace the path that data take through an entire system and then compute various timings about them such as their overall latency. Previous work on AADL (e.g., [9]) has identified a variety of different analyses that leverage flow specifications. Part of our work is identifying to what extent existing flow analyses can apply to MAPs; that is, we are investigating how they can be used to reason about local and end-to-end communication latencies, secure information

```
1  package PCA_Interlock
2  public
3  with SpO2Req_Interface, PCAPump_Interface, PCA_Interlock_Logic,
        PCA_Interlock_Display;
4    system PCA_Interlock_System
5    end PCA_Interlock_System;
6
7    system implementation PCA_Interlock_System.imp
8    subcomponents
9      spo2Device : device SpO2Req_Interface::SpO2Interface.imp;
10     appLogic : process PCA_Interlock_Logic::ICEpcaInterlockProcess.imp;
11     appDisplay : process PCA_Interlock_Display::ICEpcaDisplayProcess.imp;
12     pcaPump : device PCAPump_Interface::ICEpcaInterface.imp;
13   connections
14     -- From components to logic
15     spo2_logic : port spo2Device.SpO2 -> appLogic.SpO2;
16     DisablePump_logic : port appLogic.DisablePump -> pcaPump.DisablePump
17     {MAP_Properties::Channel_Delay => 50 ms;};
18     -- From components to display
19     spo2_disp : port spo2Device.SpO2 -> appDisplay.SpO2;
20     DisablePump_disp : port appLogic.DisablePump -> appDisplay.DisablePump;
21   flows
22     spo2_flow : end to end flow spo2Device.spo2_flow -> spo2_logic -> appLogic.
              spo2_flow -> DisablePump_logic -> pcaPump.spo2_flow;
23   end PCA_Interlock_System.imp;
24 end PCA_Interlock;
```

Fig. 4. The top-level app excerpt architecture via the AADL system component

```
1  package PCA_Interlock_Logic
2  public
3  with PCA_Interlock_Types, PCA_Interlock_Properties, MAP_Properties;
4    process ICEpcaInterlockProcess
5    features
6      SpO2 : in event data port PCA_Interlock_Types::SpO2;
7      DisablePump : out event data port PCA_Interlock_Types::Notification
8      {MAP_Properties::Output_Rate => 1 sec .. 5 sec;};
9    flows
10     spo2_flow: flow path SpO2 -> DisablePump;
11   properties
12     MAP_Properties::Component_Type => logic;
13   end ICEpcaInterlockProcess;
14
15   process implementation ICEpcaInterlockProcess.imp
16   subcomponents
17     UpdateSpO2Thread : thread UpdateSpO2Thread.imp;
18     DisablePumpThread : thread DisablePumpThread.imp;
19   connections
20     incoming_spo2 : port SpO2 -> UpdateSpO2Thread.SpO2;
21     outgoing_disable_pump : port DisablePumpThread.DisablePump -> DisablePump;
22   end ICEpcaInterlockProcess.imp;
23 end PCA_Interlock_Logic;
```

Fig. 5. An AADL process specification used in the app excerpt

flow properties, and coupling/dependencies between components of different criticality levels.

4.3 The AADL Process and Device

Now that the software and hardware elements—the AADL processes and devices marked by a ③ in Fig. 2—have been referenced by the AADL system implementation, a developer must specify their type and implementations.

AADL Processes: A process defines the boundaries of a software component, and is itself potentially composed of a number of threads (Sect. 4.4). The type of a process in AADL is a listing of that which is visible to components external to the process, i.e., the ports that other components can use to communicate with this this component (see lines 6–8 of Fig. 5). The process implementation is, like the system implementation that was discussed in Sect. 4.2, a listing of subcomponents and connections. The only valid subcomponents (in our subset of AADL) of process implementations are threads. Similarly, all connections are directional links between a thread and one of the process's ports. Both logic and display components are modeled as AADL processes, and they are distinguished from one another via the MAP_Properties::Component_Type property (line 12).

AADL Devices: Apps describe the devices they need to connect to using the AADL device construct (see Fig. 6). Device components are placeholders for actual devices that will be connected to the app when it is launched. These actual devices will have capabilities (like ports, line 6) that match the declared AADL device component specification. Note that the device implementation is left empty, since the app's device needs can be met by any device that realizes the interface requirements.

```
1  package SpO2Req_Interface
2  public
3  with PCA_Interlock_Types;
4     device SpO2Interface
5     features
6        SpO2 : out event data port PCA_Interlock_Types::SpO2;
7     flows
8        spo2_flow : flow source SpO2;
9     end SpO2Interface;
10
11    device implementation SpO2Interface.imp
12    end SpO2Interface.imp;
13 end SpO2Req_Interface;
```

Fig. 6. An AADL device used in the app excerpt

4.4 The AADL Thread

AADL threads, marked by a ④ in Fig. 2, represent semi-independent units of functionality and are realized in the MDCF as MIDAS tasks. They can be either sporadic, which signifies that they are executed when a port that they are "attached" to receives a message, or periodic, where they are executed after

```
 1  thread UpdateSpO2Thread
 2  features
 3    SpO2 : in event data port PCA_Interlock_Types::SpO2;
 4  end UpdateSpO2Thread;
 5
 6  thread implementation UpdateSpO2Thread.imp
 7  end UpdateSpO2Thread.imp;
 8
 9  thread DisablePumpThread
10  features
11    DisablePump : out event data port PCA_Interlock_Types::Notification;
12  properties
13    Thread_Properties::Dispatch_Protocol => Periodic;
14    Timing_Properties::Period => 50 ms;
15    Timing_Properties::Deadline => 10 ms;
16    Timing_Properties::Compute_Execution_Time => 5 ms;
17  end DisablePumpThread;
18
19  thread implementation DisablePumpThread.imp
20  end DisablePumpThread.imp;
```

Fig. 7. Two AADL thread interfaces used in the app excerpt

some period of time. Typically, threads which consume information operate sporadically (so they can act as soon as updated data arrive), and threads which produce information operate periodically. Alternatively, ports which are marked as data instead of event data will not trigger any thread execution, but rather will silently update a predictably-named field. This is useful in apps where there are a large number of physiological parameters; rather than specify behavior to be executed each time a message arrives, the most recent data can simply be used when needed.

Thread implementations are empty because this is the lowest level of abstraction supported; all work below this is considered "behavioral," and thus not implemented in AADL but is instead implemented within code templates auto generated by our translator. Figure 7 shows excerpts of two thread interfaces: the first consumes SpO_2 information as it arrives (lines 1–4), and the second disables the PCA pump as necessary (lines 9–17).

4.5   Concluding Tasks: Code Generation and Instantiation

At this point, the app's architecture description is complete. The next step is to generate the MAP-compatible, executable code (part (B) of Fig. 2). Our translator will interpret the AADL to create a model of the app, and then render it to a target MAP implementation; currently the only implementation supported is the MDCF. In the MDCF, Java is the language used for execution (see Fig. 8) and XML for configuration (see Fig. 9).

Execution and Configuration Code: Our app contains several components that acquire current physiological readings, others compute the conditions for shutting off the PCA pump, while others execute the interlock protocol. Figure 8 shows a very simple example of how one acquires the current SpO_2 value and

```
1  @Override
2  protected void initComponent() {
3      // TODO Fill in custom
              initialization code here
4  }
5
6  @Override
7  protected void
        SpO2ListenerOnMessage(
        MdcfMessage msg, Integer
        SpO2Data) {
8      // TODO Fill in custom listener
              code here
9  }
```

```
1  @Override
2  protected void initComponent() {
3      LatestSpO2 = -1;
4      PreviousSpO2 = -1;
5  }
6
7  @Override
8  protected void
        SpO2ListenerOnMessage(
        MdcfMessage msg, Integer
        SpO2Data) {
9      PreviousSpO2 = LatestSpO2;
10     LatestSpO2 = SpO2Data;
11 }
```

(a) Executable "skeletons" produced by the translator

(b) The same "skeletons" complete with business logic

Fig. 8. Executable code, before and after business logic implementation

```
1  <appName>PCA_Interlock_System</appName>
2  <components>
3   <VirtualComponent>
4     <name>appDisplay</name>
5     <type>ICEpcaDisplayProcess</type>
6     <role>AppPanel</role>
7   </VirtualComponent>
8   ...
9  </components>
10 <channels>
11  <Channel>
12    <chanName>$PH$</chanName>
13    <pubName>$PH$</pubName>
14    <subName>SpO2</subName>
15    <pubComp>
16      <name>$PH$</name>
17      <type>$PH$</type>
18      <role>Device</role>
19    </pubComp>
20    <subComp>
21      <name>appLogic</name>
22      <type>ICEpcaInterlockProcess</type>
23      <role>Logic</role>
24    </subComp>
25    <channelDelay>100</channelDelay>
26  </Channel>
27  ...
28 </channels>
```

```
1  <AppModuleSignature>
2   <type>ICEpcaProcess</type>
3   <moduleTasks>
4    <TaskSignature>
5     <type>PORT_SPORADIC</type>
6     <trigPort>SpO2In</trigPort>
7     <period>-1</period>
8     <name>UpdateSpO2Thread</name>
9     <deadline>50</deadline>
10    <wcetMs>5</wcetMs>
11   </TaskSignature>
12   ...
13  </moduleTasks>
14  <portSignatures>
15   <entry>
16    <string>SpO2In</string>
17    <PortSignature>
18     <name>SpO2In</name>
19     <direction>SUB</direction>
20     <minPeriod>100</minPeriod>
21     <maxPeriod>300</maxPeriod>
22     <type>Integer</type>
23    </PortSignature>
24   </entry>
25   ...
26  </portSignatures>
27 </AppModuleSignature>
```

(a) An excerpt of the app's overall layout configuration

(b) An excerpt of the logic module's configuration

Fig. 9. Configuration schemata for the app and its logic component

stores it for other components to utilize. Note that there is a great deal of auto-generated code (not shown here due to space constraints) that is hidden from the user in the development process (e.g., code for marshalling and un-marshalling messages, task instantiation, and error handling).

Figure 9a shows an excerpt of an app configuration XML file; at app launch the runtime system interprets this file and instantiates the software components. An excerpt of a software component's description is shown in Fig. 9b.

When the app is launched, the executable artifacts will combine to define the behavior of the app, and the configuration schematics will describe how the various components communicate. Part Ⓒ of Fig. 2 shows how primary elements of the app excerpt would look on an ICE implementation at runtime.

5   Conclusion

As outlined in Sect. 1, our goal for this effort was to identify "a subset of AADL that is relevant to describing the architecture of MAP applications" and to evaluate our proposal by attempting to construct a MAP app with our toolset and language. We found that while AADL was originally conceived for the aeronautics domain, it is well-suited to the description of MAP app architectures. That said, it is not a perfect fit—not only were there components whose semantics did not line up perfectly with the target domain (e.g., processes, see Sect. 4.3), but there are also predeclared properties that were defined differently than we needed. Since these properties cannot be redefined, we had to create our own (e.g., Channel_Delay). Additionally, there were port communication patterns that were only approximable with a publish-subscribe middleware (i.e., there is no shared memory access).

5.1   Future Work

As with any new proposal, we anticipate considerable iteration of our language and tooling as they mature.

Language Extensions: We are interested in considering extensions to the language to support the numerous features discussed in Sect. 2, as well as those that would enhance the rigor of the architectural descriptions consumed by our translator, such as a mechanism to specify intraprocess communication (i.e., communication between tasks in the same Java class).

Work with Collaborators: We also continue to interact with our research partners at the Center for Integration of Medicine and Innovative Technology, Underwriters Laboratories (including on the proposed UL 2800 standard for safety in medical device interoperability), and the US Food and Drug administration to validate our approach and develop guidelines for safety and regulatory reviews.

References

1. Capnostream 20 Bedside Patient Monitor. http://www.covidien.com/rms/products/capnography/capnostream-20p-bedside-patient-monitor

2. MDCF website. http://mdcf.santos.cis.ksu.edu
3. King, A., Chen, S., Lee, I.: The MIDdleware assurance substrate: enabling strong real-time guarantees in open systems with OpenFlow. In: 17th IEEE Computer Society Symposium on Object/Component/Service-Oriented Realtime Distributed Computing (ISORC 2014) (2014)
4. ASTM International. ASTM F2761 - Medical Devices and Medical Systems - Essential safety requirements for equipment comprising the patient-centric integrated clinical environment (ICE) (2009)
5. Caplan, R.A., Vistica, M.F., Posner, K.L., Cheney, F.W.: Adverse anesthetic outcomes arising from gas delivery equipment: a closed claims analysis. Anesthesiology **87**(4), 741–748 (1997)
6. Dissaux, P.: Using the aadl for mission critical software development. In: 2nd European Congress ERTS, EMBEDDED REAL TIME SOFTWARE Toulouse (2004)
7. Feiler, P.H., Gluch, D.P.: Model-Based Engineering with AADL: An Introduction to the SAE Architecture Analysis & Design Language. Addison-Wesley, Pearson (2012)
8. Feiler, P.H., Gluch, D.P., Hudak, J.J.: The architecture analysis & design language (AADL): an introduction. Technical report, DTIC Document (2006)
9. Feiler, P.H., Hansson, J.: Flow latency analysis with the architecture analysis and design language (aadl). Technical report, Carnegie Mellon University - Software Engineering Institute (2008)
10. Feiler, P.H., Hansson, J., De Niz, D., Wrage, L.: System architecture virtual integration: an industrial case study. Technical report, DTIC Document (2009)
11. Hatcliff, J., King, A., Lee, I., MacDonald, A., Fernando, A., Robkin, M., Vasserman, E., Weininger, S., Goldman, J.M.: Rationale and architecture principles for medical application platforms. In: 2012 IEEE/ACM Third International Conference on Cyber-Physical Systems (ICCPS), pp. 3–12. IEEE (2012)
12. ISO/IEEE. Domain information model. In: ISO/IEEE11073-10201 Health Informatics - Point-of-Care Medical Device Communication (2004)
13. Ivy Biomedical Systems Inc.: Vital-Guard 450C Patient Monitor with Nellcor SpO_2, August 2005
14. Kim, B., Phan, L.T., Sokolsky, O., Lee, L.: Platform-dependent code generation for embedded real-time software. In: 2013 International Conference on Compilers, Architecture and Synthesis for Embedded Systems (CASES). IEEE (2013)
15. King, A., Arney, D., Lee, I., Sokolsky, O., Hatcliff, J., Procter, S.: Prototyping closed loop physiologic control with the medical device coordination framework. In: Proceedings of the 2010 ICSE Workshop on Software Engineering in Health Care, pp. 1–11. ACM (2010)
16. King, A., Procter, S., Andresen, D., Hatcliff, J., Warren, S., Spees, W., Jetley, R., Jones, P., Weininger, S.: An open test bed for medical device integration and coordination. In: Proceedings of the 31st International Conference on Software Engineering (2009)
17. King, A.L., Procter, S., Andresen, D., Hatcliff, J., Warren, S., Spees, W., Jetley, R.P., Jones, P.L., Weininger, S.: A publish-subscribe architecture and component-based programming model for medical device interoperability. SIGBED Rev. **6**(2), 7 (2009)
18. Larson, B., Hatcliff, J., Fowler, K., Delange, J.: Illustrating the aadl error modeling annex (v. 2) using a simple safety-critical medical device. In: Proceedings of the 2013 ACM SIGAdA Annual Conference On High Integrity Language Technology, pp. 65–84. ACM (2013)

19. Larson, B., Hatcliff, J., Procter, S., Chalin, P.: Requirements specification for apps in medical application platforms. In: 2012 4th International Workshop on Software Engineering in Health Care (SEHC), pp. 26–32. IEEE (2012)
20. Maddox, R.R., Williams, C.: Clinical experience with capnography monitoring for pca patients. APSF Newsl. **26**, 3 (2012)
21. Murugesan, A., Whalen, M.W., Rayadurgam, S., Heimdahl, M.P.: Compositional verification of a medical device system. In: Proceedings of the 2013 ACM SIGAdA Annual Conference on High Integrity Language Technology. ACM (2013)
22. OSATE, S.: An extensible open source aadl tool environment. SEI AADL Team Technical report (2004)
23. Schlichting, S., Pöhlsen, S.: An architecture for distributed systems of medical devices in high acuity environments. Technical report, Dräger (2014)
24. Siegel, J.: CORBA 3 fundamentals and programming, vol. 2. Wiley, Chichester (2000)

Energy-Aware Model-Driven Development of a Wearable Healthcare Device

José Antonio Esparza Isasa[1], Peter Gorm Larsen[1(⊠)],
and Finn Overgaard Hansen[2]

[1] Department of Engineering, Aarhus University,
Finlandsgade 22, Aarhus 8200, Denmark
{jaei,pgl}@eng.au.dk
[2] Aarhus School of Engineering, Aarhus University,
Finlandsgade 22, Aarhus 8200, Denmark
foh@mail.tdcadsl.dk

Abstract. The healthcare domain is experiencing an expansion of wearable embedded devices. These devices are typically battery powered and expected to deliver a safe and reliable service to the patient regardless of its power reserves. Being energy efficient brings an additional level of complexity to the development of these solutions. In this paper we propose the application of a well-founded model-driven energy-aware approach to tackle the energy consumption in such solutions addressing all their critical subsystems: control software, communication and mechanical components. The approach enables exploration of the design space, reduces prototyping costs and helps in build confidence in the proposed solution. We demonstrate this approach in a case study focused on the development of an intelligent compression stocking to treat leg-venous insufficiency. We also discuss how this approach has benefited the development of the actual device.

Keywords: Energy consumption · Energy-aware design · Wearable devices · Pervasive healthcare · Cyber-Physical Systems

1 Introduction

Wearable embedded systems are a concrete kind of Cyber-Physical Systems (CPSs) that are experiencing a widespread application in the healthcare domain. Given their nature these devices are mainly battery powered and present a challenge from the *sustainability* point of view. Additionally the medical domain adds *safety* and *security* constraints during their operation. These properties are know as the S3 properties of CPSs [2], they are common to many other systems but specially relevant in medical CPSs. Being energy efficient as well as satisfying the functional requirements is a complex challenge when designing these kinds of devices. The application of abstract modelling at the system level to cope with this complexity has been proposed [8]. These models enable the analysis

© Springer International Publishing AG 2017
M. Huhn and L. Williams (Eds.): FHIES 2014/SEHC 2014, LNCS 9062, pp. 44–63, 2017.
DOI: 10.1007/978-3-319-63194-3_4

of system properties and they can be progressively transformed into concrete system realizations. This approach is know as model-driven development.

We propose a new way to conduct energy-aware model-driven development of complex embedded solutions, enabling the analysis of energy consumption from different perspectives: communication, computation and electro-mechanical [13]. In this paper we present how we have applied this approach to the design of a medical-grade intelligent compression stocking in order to study energy consumption and steer the development of the device. The application of this approach has resulted in the redesign of the mechanical configuration and control software leading to energy savings of up to 33%. Additionally we have explored several system architectures involving software and hardware at the modelling level, being able to choose the optimal one for the current implementation.

The remainder of this paper is structured as follows: Sect. 2 gives an overview of the modelling approach applied to the design of a concrete healthcare device, which is presented in Sect. 3. Section 4 ellaborates on the results achieved so far. Sections 5 and 6 present related and future work respectively. Finally, Sect. 7 concludes this paper.

2 Energy-Aware Model-Driven Design

CPSs are complex systems composed of electro-mechanical, software, electronic and communication components. We propose the application of a heterogeneous modelling approach, that incorporates the notion of consumed energy, to take all these elements into consideration in a single design effort [13]. This section introduces the modelling technologies used and outlines this approach.

2.1 Modelling Technologies Used

Given the heterogeneous composition of a CPS we have used two different modelling paradigms that can be used cooperatively to develop systems. These paradigms are used to represent the system and to some extent the interaction with the environment through Discrete Event and Continuous Time models. The tools supporting them are:

Overture[1]: is a modelling environment that supports the creation and simulation of VDM Real-Time models [16,22]. This formal notation is suitable for the representation of Discrete Event (DE) control logic. It supports the deployment of different model parts on different simulated CPUs that are connected by buses. This makes it possible to simulate some of the distributed properties of a CPS.

20-Sim[2]: is a modelling environment that supports the creation of Continuous Time (CT) models based on differential equations. Additionally it incorporates higher level abstractions such as bond graphs and libraries of ready

---

[1] Overture project official website: www.overturetool.org.
[2] 20-sim official website www.20sim.com.

made components for different areas (pneumatics, electronics and hydraulics among others).

DESTECS/Crescendo[3]: is a framework that connects the Overture real time interpreter with the simulation core of 20-Sim [3,6]. This provides a common notion of time for both simulators and makes it possible to run them in parallel with interactions (co-simulation) [7].

These tools are general purpose modelling tools within their respective domains, that can be used to study different system functionalities not necessarily involving energy consumption. For additional details on the tools and how they can be applied refer to [6] and continuations of this work in the INTO-CPS[4] project [4,5,18,19].

2.2 Model-Based Approach to Energy Consumption

Our design approach [13] takes into consideration energy consumption in systems from three different angles: mechanical, software and communication.

Mechanical Modelling. Mechanical components incorporated in a CPS are typically the most energy consuming ones. These mechanical and electro-mechanical components are controlled from software and typically feature different kinds of sensors and actuators. Ways to decrease their energy consumption include the design of new mechanical architectures or the optimization of control algorithms. This implies that one needs to consider both electro-mechanics and control logic together in order to find an energy efficient system configuration. An example of an electro-mechanical subsystem in a wearable healthcare device could be the components responsible for a blood pressure measurement in a pervasive blood pressure measurement monitor (i.e., inflatable cuff, pump, manometer and valves).

Electro-mechanical devices are best modelled using CT abstractions such as differential equations and this makes the application of 20-Sim suitable in this case. On the other hand the control logic behind these components is best represented using DE abstractions such as VDM-RT. We use Crescendo in order to enable collaborative simulation making it possible to simulate complex control logic represented in VDM-RT with accurate physical models created under 20-sim. We proposed a particular way of applying this technology so energy consumption can be taken into account and one can perform trade-off analysis among different candidate solutions [10].

---

[3] This framework is currently known as Crescendo but it was called DESTECS in previous published work (see www.crescendotool.org).

[4] This is an acronym for "Integrated Tool Chain for Model-based Design of Cyber-Physical Systems" and information can be found at www.into-cps.au.dk.

Software Modelling. Energy consumption caused by software execution can be quantified at different levels of abstraction ranging from the microarchitectural level all the way up the operating systems services. We have analyzed it from a development point of view, in which a system designer can decide for how long and when the software execution can be halted and the processing core put in a low-power sleeping mode. Such a mode is supported by most of today's microcontrollers and the way it is used can have a significant impact on energy consumption. We propose the application of the VDM-RT modelling language to study how different sleeping policies can be used in the system. VDM-RT is appropriate in this case because it can represent control logic using a DE paradigm. Additionally it provides a virtual execution environment through the CPU abstraction, which we have extended so it is able to be put to sleep and activated through specific operations [11]. Regarding the case of the pervasive blood pressure measurement, an example of software in a healthcare device could be the logic that determines when a measurement has to be conducted and detects abnormal patient conditions.

Communication Modelling. Energy consumption on the communication side as in the software case can be studied at different levels of abstraction. We focus our study on characterizing the usage of the network interface (for instance 802.15.4 or Bluetooth Low Energy (BLE) radio) in terms of mode of operation and duration. This analysis can be conducted to some extent with the VDM-RT modelling language thanks to its ability to model distributed aspects [17]. VDM-RT incorporates the abstraction BUS, that is used to connect different CPU execution environments. We proposed specific ways in which this can be used to represent small scale network topologies and how the notion of energy can be incorporated to it [13].

An example of a communication subsystem following the previous example of pervasive blood pressure measurements could be a Blueetooth Low Energy radio that allows this device to be part of a Body Area Network for patient monitoring.

Even though we have used the formal notation VDM-RT to represent software related aspects, we have not conducted formal verification over the models. The validation of the models has been conducted purely through simulation. The rationale behind this approach is to be able to explore the design space in a cost effective way. Since VDM-RT is used to represent the system it can be possible sometime in the future to conduct formal verification.

3   Design of an Intelligent Medical Grade Compression Stocking

In order to analyze the validity of our approach we have applied these techniques to a concrete, real case study. This case study is based on the European Ambient Assisted Living project e-Stocking, in which we are creating an intelligent compression stocking to treat leg-venous insufficiency[5]. This system is

---

[5] e-Stockings project official website: http://www.e-stockings.eu/.

required to deliver a compression that ranges from 40 mmHg at the ankle level to 20 mmHg below the knee. This wearable healthcare device is composed of mechanical, software and communication subsystems and since it is a medical device it must conform to a high level of quality. The device can be seen in Fig. 1. This compression principle is based on three different inflatable bladders. The system consists of a set of pumps and a valve, an embedded control unit, a radio communication interface and a battery. A complete description of this system can be found in [15].

3.1 Design Challenges

The main design challenges to be addressed during the development of this device are:

- The operational time should be between 12 to 14 hours, enabling the patient a complete day of use without requiring a battery recharge.
- The pressure delivered to the limb shall be constant and within the prescribed range. This implies that the stocking shall feature a regulation mechanism that makes sure that the delivered compression is inside the specified interval.
- The stocking controller should be able to communicate with a smartphone acting as an internet gateway and/or a configuration tool.

We aim to tackle these challenges to some extent through the application of our modelling approach by: gaining a better understanding of the problem and being able to provide solution candidates based on the Design Space Exploration (DSE) conducted through modelling.

3.2 Component Power Consumption

The stocking system is composed of components of very different nature with different power consumption figures across different orders of magnitude. In order to give a better overview of the subsystem power consumptions we present the power requirements[6] of the key components of the system in Table 1.

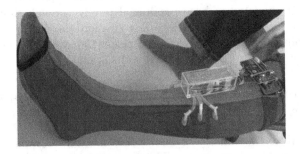

Fig. 1. The e-Stocking prototype.

---

[6] These figures should be considered as average and approximate within their respective order of magnitude.

Table 1. Overview of the typical components power consumption:

Component	Current draw	Voltage	Power consumption
Pump	110 mA	3 V	330 mW
Valve	120 mA	3 V	360 mW
Manometers	1.4 mA	3.3 V	4.62 mW
CPU Active/Sleeping/Hibernating	20 mA/10 uA/10 nA	3.3 V	66 mW/33 uW/33 nW
Radio Tx/Rx	35/40 mA	3.3 V	115.5/132 mW

Inspection of these figures reveals that electromechanical components such as pump and valves are the most power demanding. Since these are heavily used to administer the compression, initial efforts to minimize energy consumption should be focused in the mechanical area.

3.3 Mechanical Co-modelling

The mechanical side (also know as a *plant* in the control engineering domain) of the compression stocking has been represented in a 20-sim CT model. The plant control logic has been modelled in VDM-RT. The combination of the two models has been co-simulated using Crescendo. An overview of the mechanical side is given in Fig. 2 and its components are described below.

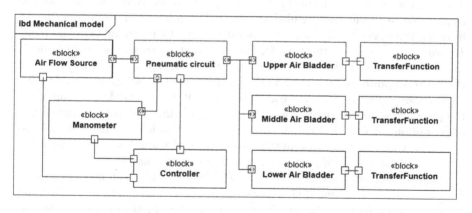

Fig. 2. SysML Internal Block Diagram of the mechanical model.

Air Flow Source: represents the pump that generates the air flow to be directed to the air-bladders to build pressure. It is controlled by the software controller and the effective airflow can be modulated.

Pneumatic Circuit: represents a concrete arrangement of valves and tubing connections. The valves are controllable from the software and this makes it possible to direct the air-flow to a single air bladder. The valves are also responsible for the venting of the air bladders, however this cannot be modulated.

Manometer: is an air pressure sensor that can monitor the level of compression in the different air bladders. Due to the way it is connected through the pneumatic circuit a single manometer can be used to monitor any of the three chambers.

Air Bladders: represent the chambers integrated in the stocking in which pressure builds-up. Their air intake can be locked without having to energized the valves.

Transfer Functions: are different mathematical expressions that determine how the pressure in the air chambers map to the pressure over the skin, representing the effective compression. They can be replaced depending on the compression principle under evaluation and the rest of the model still can be reused.

Controller: contains the necessary interface definitions to communicate the mechanical model with the software control logic modelled in VDM-RT.

Figure 3 presents the top level representation of the 20-sim plant model. The complete model connects two more bladder subsystems (shown with the dashed box) to the distribution valve, but they have been removed in this case for clarity. The pneumatic circuit presented above is decomposed in a *Distribution valve* and one *Pass valve* per bladder subsystem. The *Distribution valve* is responsible for directing the air flow to the air bladder that has to be inflated. The *Pass valve* is responsible for locking the air bladder once inflation has been completed. Hence, in order to inflate an air bladder two valves have to be energized. The block *LegSegment* introduced the transfer function that maps the pressure built in the *AirBladders* with the pressure exerted over the leg. This model incorporates the notion of power consumption in the most power demanding components: the *Distribution valve*, the *Pass valve* and the *Pump*. When the models are simulated the power consumption figures are integrated over time, resulting in the energy consumption for each individual component. The models are instrumented so both power and energy consumption are monitored variables in the simulation but without having an impact on the simulation performance.

The software controller modelled in VDM-RT contains the necessary interfaces to control the simulated sensors (manometer) and actuators (valve and pump). Additionally it features different regulation algorithms and configurations. These regulation algorithms aim at maintaining the pressure in the air bladders constant and constitute the core logic of the DE models. The most relevant ones are:

Simple regulation: that is based on conditional logical statements and do not modulate the pump air flow. This implies that the pump will be engaged fully in case additional compression is needed and the air bladders will be vented in case over-pressure occurs.

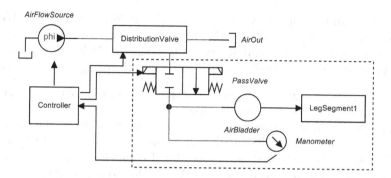

Fig. 3. 20-sim CT model of the compression stocking.

PID regulation: Proportional Integral Derivative [24], that modulates the pump airflow depending on the deviation from the target pressure. Due to this behaviour it is said to be proportional in the inflation. Due to the mechanical construction of the system it is not possible to modulate the venting process and therefore it cannot be made proportional in the deflation. Therefore, a full PID controller cannot be incorporated in this system.

Listing 1 shows part of the model for a proportional regulation of the pressure in one of the air bladders. In this case the pump is driven proportionally to the error (err): the difference between current and target pressure (setPoint). Prior to engage the pump at specific rate, the controller sets the air distribution valve and opens the pass valve for the target air bladder (AB1).

```
err := setPoint - manometerAB1.getPressure();
if (err > threshold) then (
  pTerm = err * pGain;
  controller.airDistribution.airToAB1();
  controller.passValveAB1.open();
  controller.pump.setPumpRate(pTerm); );
```

Listing 1. Proportional regulation applied to air bladder 1.

The execution of these models has enabled us to explore different regulation configurations to determine their effectiveness as well as to compare them regarding their energy performance. We evaluated two different scenarios: compression from an idle state and regulation after an under-pressure event occurred. Such an event might happen due to small leaks that have an impact on the pressure level during treatment. The simulation of the models allowed us to draw the following conclusions:

– The energy consumption during inflation and regulation is proportional to the time this process has taken and this is due to the particular configuration of the pneumatic circuit.

- This time can be reduced by inflating the air bladders as fast as possible, by configuring the PID controller with a high proportional constant,
- This implies that the valves that have to be triggered during inflation will be energized as briefly as possible, hence decreasing the energy consumption.

Applying this principle to the design of the software controller has lead to a decrement of $\approx 33\%$ in energy consumption.

Additionally we have been able to explore ways to stabilize the controller taking into consideration different PID configurations. Given the fact that only the inflation can be controlled in a proportional manner and not the deflation, this has turned to be a challenging task. We decided to apply an error window that determines whether or not the regulation must be executed (hysteresis). This window should be taken into account in order to determine the periodicity of the regulation logic. A higher error window would result on a higher period for the real time thread that executes the controller. This could have an impact on the way the software makes use of the computational resources and therefore in the energy consumption. This is discussed further in the section below.

3.4 Software Modelling

The control regulation logic introduced in the previous section is deployed as a software component, executed by the CPU integrated on the e-Stocking micro-controller. This CPU features a number of low power operational states to choose between when developing applications. Depending on the low power state used by the developer (Sleeping or Hibernating[7]) different kinds of wake-up mechanisms are available. In this work we have considered the following and most common ones:

Wake-up on sleep timer expiration: The CPU remains in a low power state until an internal timer overflows, generating an internal (within the chip) interrupt that wakes up the CPU. Applying this wake-up mechanism typically implies using the more energy demanding low power states such as the Sleep mode.

Wake-up on external event: The CPU remains in a low power state until an external event generates an interrupt that activates it. Applying this wake-up mechanism allow the use of Sleep or Hibernation modes.

These mechanisms facilitate the implementation of two different software regulation strategies for the e-Stocking case study:

Periodic regulation: in which the regulation logic is executed as a periodic thread. The period that determines how often the logic has to be executed can

---

[7] Modern CPUs incorporate several low power modes, the most common being: a *Sleep* mode with a current draw within the order of microamps and a *Hibernation* mode, with a current draw of nanoamps and less reactive than the first one. Mode names vary depending on the manufacturer.

be determined by the study of the control requirements carried out during the mechanical modelling, presented in the section above. While the regulation is not executing, the processor can be put to sleep. This approach makes use of a *Wake-up on sleep timer expiration* strategy.

Event-triggered regulation: in which the regulation logic is executed once a pressure loss has been detected by smart sensors. The CPU can be put to sleep for an undefined period of time and remain in that state until it is notified by any of the sensors. This approach makes use of a *Wake-up on external event* strategy.

The energy consumption will depend directly on the strategy adopted and how it uses the low power features based on sleeping modes. These regulation strategies are implemented through two different system architectures, shown in the UML deployment diagram presented in Fig. 4. These architectures are:

Architecture A: implements a periodic regulation strategy in which the CPU executes regulation logic and moves to sleeping state. After the sleep timer has expired it wakes up the CPU and executes the regulation process again. The system uses passive pressure sensors that have to be actively polled by the CPU.

Architecture B: implements an aperiodic regulation strategy in which the CPU hibernates until an abnormal pressure level is detected by the pressure sensors. This architecture makes use of Smart Pressure sensors, capable of monitoring the pressure levels independently of the main CPU. Once a pressure deviation has been detected by these pressure sensors they generate an external interrupt that wake up the main CPU, that will finally execute the regulation logic. The power consumption of these sensors is higher than the passive sensors but still negligible and orders of magnitude below the power consumption of the CPU executing the control logic.

Common to both architectures are the CPU core and the PWMDriver block, that is responsible for generating the airflow to inflate the chambers.

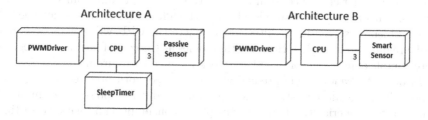

Fig. 4. Deployment diagram with architectures for the two different regulation strategies.

Both architectures have been modelled in VDM-RT as shown in the deployment diagram presented in Fig. 5. In this diagram we use nodes to represent the

VDM-RT CPUs (stereotyped as <<CPU>>). In these CPUs we deploy different parts of the model to run independently and they are connected through
VDM-RT BUSes. This model can be configured in two different ways to represent either Architecture A or B, by using the model of the SleepTimer or the
WakeUpInterrupt respectively. The Controller class deployed in the node
mcu models the logic that implements the regulation functionality presented in
the previous Listing 1 as well as the logic that determines whether the CPU is
sleeping or not.

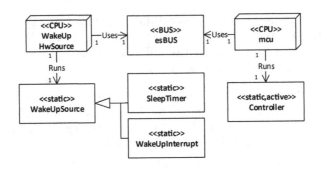

Fig. 5. Class diagram showing the models general structure.

We simulated these two architectures under a common scenario in which we
considered the regulation over a period of time of 200 ms. In this scenario we
simulated a pressure loss taking place at 150 ms. We simulated both system models and represented their power consumption over time, producing the activity
graphs shown in Fig. 6. Based on these CPU activity graphs, taking into consideration CPU manufacturer specifications and basic CPU current draw measurements we were able to predict concrete average power and energy consumption
figures.

The simulation of these models show that the software used in Architecture A
results in a higher energy consumption, since it causes periodic unnecessary system wake-ups to check pressure levels even though the regulation is not needed.
This problem is solved in Architecture B where the CPU will not be activated
until a regulation is needed. However this comes at the cost of having to integrate
more complex smart sensors[8], able to work independently from the CPU.

In order to validate our predictions we realized both architectures, implemented both regulation strategies and measured their power consumption.
Finally, after numerically integrating the power consumption measured over time
we determined the total energy consumption. The energy consumption predicted
differed from the actual energy consumption by less than 5%. The measurements
conducted over the two concrete system realizations are presented in Fig. 7. Due

---

[8] The power consumption of these sensors is not taken into consideration because it
is negligible if compared with the power consumption of the CPU.

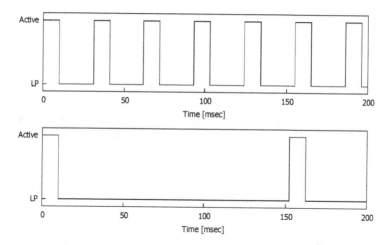

Fig. 6. Activity over time predicted by the models in Architectures A (upper graph) and B (lower graph) in the scenario under study.

to the specifics of the processor used in the prototype (ARM Cortex M3) it was possible to use a hibernation mode in the implementation of architecture B. Such a mode has lower current draw than the sleep mode (four orders of magnitude below). This is reflected in the measurements presented in Fig. 7.

This initial application of modelling to energy consumption on the software side shows that our approach is sufficiently accurate to validate at the abstract modelling level computation issues from the power and energy consumption point of view.

Additionally it is worthwhile remarking that the same kind of analysis can be conducted with any software functionality running on the systems CPU that might have an impact on energy consumption. Obvious candidates for further analysis would be communication software and security protocols.

3.5   Communication Modelling

The e-Stocking case present several communication scenarios [9]. We have focused on the most relevant from the energy consumption point of view:

Health monitoring: In this scenario the stocking transmits current and historical data regarding treatment adherence and condition evolution.
Calibration and configuration: In this scenario the stocking settings that determine how the treatment is conducted (mainly pressure levels) are set through an external device.

In order to model these scenarios, we proposed the application of the Distributed Real-Time features of VDM-RT. The models developed using VDM-RT follow the structure presented in [13]. This structure supports the modelling

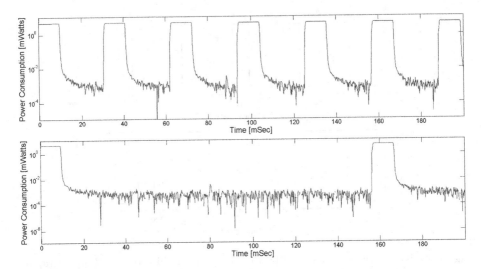

Fig. 7. Actual power consumption of the control logic execution over time in Architectures A (upper graph) and B (lower graph). Note the logarithmic vertical scale

of small-scale networks such as Body Area Networks with several nodes interacting. In this case this structure can be simplified since there are only two nodes communicating. This structure is applied to this case as shown in the UML deployment diagram presented in Fig. 8. The resulting model uses VDM-RT CPUs as execution environments in which the communication logic is run. The nodes represent the e-Stocking and an external client that connects to it in order to perform Health monitoring or Calibration and configuration as described above. The connection between the two nodes is represented through a VDM-RT BUS representing a 802.154 link. Each node is able to transmit data to the other by pushing it through the bus to the target receive buffer (`eSBuffer` and `clientBuffer`). Each node is able to receive data by reading its local receive buffers.

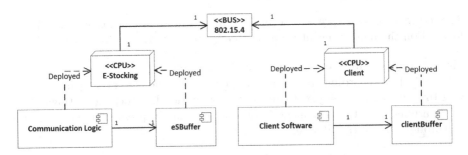

Fig. 8. UML deployment diagram showing the structure of the VDM-RT communication models.

The modelling approach we have followed to study communication is composed of the following steps:

1. **Abstract protocol modelling (Model 1):** consists of high level modelling
   of the communication process, capturing the interactions between the devices.
   These models represent the information exchanged by tokens. No notion of
   energy is present at this stage.
2. **Definition of application level messages (Model 2):** consist on the
   creation of the application level Protocol Data Units (PDU) that will be
   exchanged between the devices. These messages can be made part of the
   model and replace the tokens.
3. **Profiling of the communication interface power consumption:** this
   is the characterization of the network interface used to communciate the
   devices. This profiling can be made experimentally or by consulting the product datasheets. As a result of this step it should be possible to have a rather
   precise estimation of the transmission and reception power consumption per
   byte.
4. **Profiling energy consumption of each message exchanged in the
   communication:** this is the construction of a look-up table in which it is
   described how much energy it takes to send and receive each message that
   compose the protocol.
5. **Model execution and production of energy consumption estimations (Model 3):** results on a high-fidelity energy consumption estimation
   based on the previous models capturing the interactions and the characterization of the energy consumption of each package exchange.
6. **Protocol rework:** in case it is desired one can rework the interactions or
   the protocol in order to lower the power consumption of the communication.

The initial abstract model captures the interactions between the client and
the e-stocking in terms of who is initiating the communication and what information is exchanged. The communication logic executed in each party is modelled in separate procedural threads handling the communication buffers. Initially these models do not make use of the notion of time present in VDM-RT
since communication-related times have not been determined yet. Taking as an
example the configuration scenario and focusing on the communication in the
e-Stocking node, we can see the output of such a model in the first column of
Table 2.

After this initial modeling, and following step two of our communication
modelling approach, we defined the application level messages that correspond
to the tokens used previously. This gives a better idea regarding the amount of
information that has to be exchanged between the client and the stocking. The
results of this modelling step are shown as an addition to model execution log
shown before in Table 2, column 2.

Once these modelling stages were completed we proceed to study the communication interface power consumption during transmission and reception. We
determine the power consumption of the interface in transmission and reception

Table 2. e-Stocking communication model execution results for the configuration scenario:

Model 1 Interactions	Model 2 Information	Model 3 Time, energy consumption
< − − RX <ConnectionRequest>	s0e	0.5 ms +22 µJ
− − >TX <ACK>	s1e	1 ms +64 µJ
< − − RX <SetPressures>	s53203040e	1.5 ms +22 µJ
− − >TX <ACK>	s1e	
		2 ms +64 µJ
< − − RX <Disconnection>	s2e	2.5 ms +22 µJ
Total communication time 2.5 ms, Total energy consumption: 194 µJ		

experimentally and based on these measurements determined the energy consumed per transmitted and received message. Due to the extra headers added by layers underneath the application, the high baudrate of the communication link, and similar application message lenghts, there is very small difference among the messages considered in terms of transmissions and receptions times and, therefore, in power consumption. Figure 9 shows the power consumption in the communication interface when transmitting and receiving a single byte.

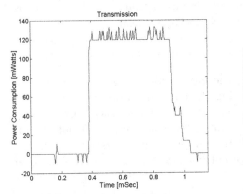 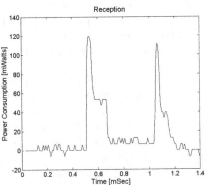

Fig. 9. Power consumption for a single byte transmission and reception in the communication interface.

After gaining insight into the physical implications in the communication interface of different kinds of messages, it is possible to establish real transmission and reception times as well as real power consumption figures. This makes it possible to incorporate the measurements to the communication models and create high fidelity estimations in terms of communication times and communication energy consumption. The final models are able to produce extended logs in which time and energy are taken into account. Table 2 shows the extended model execution results in column 3.

Besides analyzing the configuration scenario, we have also studied the health monitoring scenario. In this case we have proceed in a similar manner, following the steps defined previously, with the only difference that we decided to rework the communication logic, sending longer messages containing more information to minimize the energy spent on transmitting headers.

4   Results and Discussion

The creation of the initial mechanical model already had a positive impact on the development process without taking energy consumption into consideration. This preliminary model helped us in getting an understanding of the pneumatics domain before delving into particular implementation aspects. Regarding the particular case study, through the modelling of the mechanical subsystem it became clear that establishing a transfer function that determined how pressure inside the air bladders mapped to the skin was critical to achieve an effective regulation. This led to the incorporation of a manometer into the system to enable measurements of air pressure in the system. Both suggestions have been transferred to the real implementation of the system being carried out in parallel. Additionally, through the application of modelling we were able to evaluate an alternative compression mechanism and discard it since it was not a feasible solution. The same conclusion was reached by a partner working in parallel but through prototyping.

Regarding energy consumption in computation, other approaches to energy savings apply dynamic frequency and voltages scaling. Such an approach is not especially helpful in this case because the operations carried out during the regulation are not especially computationally intensive. Additionally there is a bottleneck time-wise in the interaction with the physical environment (such as the sensor's response time). Finally, there are very small variations between different operating frequencies in the CPU used and therefore one cannot save as much energy as in the current approach through the application of sleeping operational modes.

The estimates that we were able to achieve through the application of modelling in this case study were coarse grained estimates, fit for the purpose of facilitating taking design decisions and trade-off analysis. For more precise figures (especially in the mechanical case) it is necessary to perform concrete measurements on the concrete realization.

The application of models has allowed us to conduct DSE without having to conduct extensive prototyping of several solutions and without having to run long batches of experiments manually. This brings the advantage of reduced costs in system development due to lesser expenditures in development time and prototyping material.

This approach to system design would be ideally carried out by at least two engineers: one with a thorough knowledge of mechanics and physical modelling and a second expert in embedded systems, including both hardware and software issues. Experts in embedded systems typically have certain knowledge of system communications and therefore can also cover energy consumption on that side. In our case this methodology has been applied by a single engineer specialized in the embedded area but with a basic knowledge of pneumatics. Occasional support on mechanical modelling was provided by experts on the field. The modelling conducted by this single engineer resulted in several design suggestions and input to the development of the compression stocking being carried out in parallel. From an industrial perspective developers who wishes to use a similar approach would need to learn the different modelling notations. Given that you understand the underlying theory that is not hard but as with any other technology "A fool with a tool is still a fool", so there is no doubt that there is a modest investment in how to model things sufficiently accurate so the models get competent.

5   Related Work

The energy consumption in CPS in general and in wearable devices is a well recognized problem [2,23]. Typical approaches to wearable healthcare systems are based on the development of prototypes. Extensive examples of systems developed following this approach can be found in the literature (e.g. [20,25]). However, these approaches are purely focused on system functionality rather than energy efficiency and therefore they address it at the end of the development process and as a final factor to optimize. Opposed to this prototyping-based methodology one can only find limited related work in which a model-driven approach is applied to the development wearable healthcare systems. Anliker et. al. propose a concrete method to design distributed wearable systems, making special emphasis on the analysis of computation and communication logic [1]. This approach considers energy consumption among other design factors and they formalize them through the application of different metrics to perform DSE. Previous modelling work exists on wearable health monitoring devices through Stochastic Petri Nets [21]. This work is very focused on the software functionality and does not take energy consumption into consideration.

Finally, the development of wearable healthcare devices can benefit from some of the model-based approaches to CPS design, such as the one shown in DESTECS [3] and presented before the one proposed by Jensen et al. [14]. Even though these do not make special emphasis on the energy consumption of the system, the provided tools that can be used following the approach we proposed in [13] so energy consumption can be taken into account during the development process and described from different perspectives.

6   Future Work

The analysis conducted in this case study has enabled the production of energy consumption estimations by conducting simple initial measurements combined with modelling. At this point we are considering how this model-based engineering approach can benefit from partial system prototyping. This could potentially be facilitated by our previous work in Hardware in the Loop and the combination of models and partial system realizations in a single co-execution [12]. Additionally we are applying the same energy-aware model-driven engineering approach discussed in here to a second case study in the medical domain: a platform for The Pacemaker Formal Methods Challenge[9], paying especial attention to the energy consumption analysis.

7 Conclusion

We have presented the application of an energy-aware model-based approach to the development of a wearable medical device: a compression stocking to treat leg-venous insufficiency. This approach has taken into consideration three critical subsystems that compose this solution: mechanical, computation and communication subsystems. The modelling techniques presented here combined with partial prototyping have helped us during the analysis, design and implementation of this compression stocking. Thanks to the application of modelling we have been able to evaluate different mechanical compression principles, redesign mechanical subsystem to reduce energy consumption, evaluate different regulation algorithms and get a grasp on how the software can be configured to reduce energy consumption. Additionally we have evaluated the energy consumption in different communication scenarios.

Hopefully this work will inspire other medical device developers and convince them to apply a model-based approach instead of a prototyping-driven one, allowing them to gain confidence on the solution designed and to reduce development costs.

Acknowledgements. This research is partially funded by the EU Ambient Assisted Living Joint Programme, eStockings Project under grant agreement no. AAL-2011-4-020.

References

1. Anliker, U., Beutel, J., Dyer, M., et al.: A systematic approach to the design of distributed wearable systems. IEEE Trans. Comput. **53**(8), 1017–1033 (2004)
2. Banerjee, A., Venkatasubramanian, K.K., Mukherjee, T., Gupta, S.K.S.: Ensuring safety, security, and sustainability of mission-critical cyber-physical systems. Proc. IEEE **100**(1), 283–299 (2012)
3. Broenink, J.F., Larsen, P.G., Verhoef, M., Kleijn, C., Jovanovic, D., Pierce, K., Wouters, F.: Design support and tooling for dependable embedded control software. In: Proceedings of Serene 2010 International Workshop on Software Engineering for Resilient Systems, pp. 77–88. ACM, April 2010

---

[9] More details can be found in http://sqrl.mcmaster.ca/pacemaker.htm.

4. Fitzgerald, J., Gamble, C., Larsen, P.G., Pierce, K., Woodcock, J.: Cyber-physical systems design: formal foundations, methods and integrated tool chains. In: FormaliSE: FME Workshop on Formal Methods in Software Engineering, Florence, Italy, May 2015, ICSE 2015 (2015)
5. Fitzgerald, J., Gamble, C., Payne, R., Larsen, P.G., Basagiannis, S., Mady, A.E.-D.: Collaborative model-based systems engineering for cyber-physical systems - a case study in building automation. In: INCOSE 2016, Edinburgh, Scotland, July 2016
6. Fitzgerald, J., Larsen, P.G., Verhoef, M. (eds.): Collaborative Design for Embedded Systems - Co-modelling and Co-simulation. Springer, Heidelberg (2014). doi:10.1007/978-3-642-54118-6
7. Gomes, C., Thule, C., Broman, D., Larsen, P.G., Vangheluwe, H.: Co-simulation: state of the art. Technical report, February 2017
8. Gupta, S.K.S., Mukherjee, T., Varsamopoulos, G., Banerjee, A.: Research directions in energy-sustainable cyberphysical systems. Sustain. Comput. Inf. Syst. 1(1), 57–74 (2011)
9. Hansen, F.O., Jensen, T.F., Esparza, J.A.: Distributed ICT architecture for developing, configuring and monitoring mobile embedded healthcare systems. In: International Conference on Health Informatics (HEALTHINF 2014), March 2014
10. Isasa, J.A.E., Hansen, F.O., Larsen, P.G.: Embedded systems energy consumption analysis through co-modelling and simulation. In: Proceedings of the International Conference on Modeling and Simulation, ICMS 2013. World Academy of Science, Engineering and Technology, June 2013
11. Isasa, J.A.E., Jørgensen, P.W.V., Ballegaard, C.: Modelling energy consumption in embedded systems with VDM-RT. In: Proceedings of the 4th International ABZ Conference, July 2014
12. Isasa, J.A.E., Jørgensen, P.W.V., Larsen, P.G.: Hardware in the loop for VDM-real time modelling of embedded systems. Hardware in the loop for VDM-real time modelling of embedded systems. In: MODELSWARD 2014, Second International Conference on Model-Driven Engineering and Software Development, January 2014
13. Isasa, J.A.E., Larsen, P.G., Hansen, F.O.: A holistic approach to energy-aware design of cyber-physical systems. Int. J. Embed. Syst. 9(3), 283–295 (2017)
14. Jensen, J.C., Chang, D.H., Lee, E.A.: A model-based design methodology for cyber-physical systems. In: 7th International Wireless Communications and Mobile Computing Conference (IWCMC), pp. 1666–1671 (2011)
15. Jensen, T.F., Hansen, F.O., Isasa, J.A.E., et al.: ICT-enabled medical compression stocking for treatment of leg-venous insufficiency. In: International Conference on Biomedical Electronics and Devices (BIODEVICES 2014), March 2014
16. Battle, N.N., Ferreira, M., Fitzgerald, J., Lausdahl, K., Verhoef, M.: The overture initiative - integrating tools for VDM. SIGSOFT Softw. Eng. 35(1), 1–6 (2010)
17. Larsen, P.G., Fitzgerald, J.S., Wolff, S.: Methods for the development of distributed real-time embedded systems using VDM. Int. J. Softw. Inform. 3(2–3), 305–341 (2009)
18. Larsen, P.G., Fitzgerald, J., Woodcock, J., Fritzson, P., Brauer, J., Kleijn, C., Lecomte, T., Pfeil, M., Green, O., Basagiannis, S., Sadovykh, A.: Integrated tool chain for model-based design of cyber-physical systems: the INTO-CPS project. In: CPS Data Workshop, Vienna, Austria (2016)
19. Larsen, P. G., Fitzgerald, J., Woodcock, J., Lecomte, T.: Collaborative modelling and simulation for cyber-physical systems In: Trustworthy Cyber-Physical Systems Engineering. Chapman and Hall/CRC, September 2016. ISBN 9781498742450

20. Mokhlespour, M.I., Zobeiri, O., Narimani, R., et al.: Design and Prototyping of wearable measuring system for trunk movement using textile sensors. In: Proceedings of the 20th Iranian Conference on Electrical Engineering, (ICEE 2012), pp. 1571–1575, May 2012

21. Pantelopoulos, A., Bourbakis, N.: SPN-model based simulation of a wearable health monitoring system. In: Proceedings of the 31st Annual International Conference of the IEEE EMBS, pp. 320–323. IEEE, September 2009

22. Verhoef, M., Larsen, P.G., Hooman, J.: Modeling and validating distributed embedded real-time systems with VDM++. In: Misra, J., Nipkow, T., Sekerinski, E. (eds.) FM 2006. LNCS, vol. 4085, pp. 147–162. Springer, Heidelberg (2006). doi:10.1007/11813040_11

23. Vuorela, T.: Technologies for wearable and portable physiological measurement devices. PhD thesis, Tampere University of Technology (2011)

24. Wescott, T.: PID without a PhD. Embed. Syst. Des. **13**, 86–108 (2000)

25. Wong, K.-I.: Rapid prototyping of a low-power, wireless, reflectance photoplethysmography system. In: Proceedings of the 2010 International Conference on Body Sensor Networks, pp. 47–51 (2010)

Reasoning About Confidence
and Uncertainty in Assurance Cases: A Survey

Lian Duan[1(✉)], Sanjai Rayadurgam[1], Mats P.E. Heimdahl[1],
Anaheed Ayoub[2], Oleg Sokolsky[2], and Insup Lee[2]

[1] University of Minnesota, Minneapolis, USA
{lduan,rsanjai,heimdahl}@cs.umn.edu
[2] University of Pennsylvania, Philadelphia, USA
aae.anaheed@gmail.com, {sokolsky,lee}@cis.upenn.edu

Abstract. Assurance cases are structured logical arguments supported
by evidence that explain how systems, possibly software systems, satisfy desirable properties for safety, security or reliability. The confidence
in both the logical reasoning and the underlying evidence is a factor
that must be considered carefully when evaluating an assurance case;
the developers must have confidence in their case before the system is
delivered and the assurance case reviewer, such as a regulatory body,
must have adequate confidence in the case before approving the system for use. A necessary aspect of gaining confidence in the assurance
case is dealing with uncertainty, which may have several sources. Uncertainty, often impossible to eliminate, nevertheless undermines confidence
and must therefore be sufficiently bounded. It can be broadly classified
into two types, *aleatory* (statistical) and *epistemic* (systematic). This
paper surveys how researchers have reasoned about uncertainty in assurance cases. We analyze existing literature to identify the type of uncertainty addressed and distinguish between qualitative and quantitative
approaches for dealing with uncertainty.

1 Introduction

Systems developed for medical, transportation, and infrastructure applications
that significantly impact life, property, or environment typically need to gain the
approval of an independent entity such as a regulatory body. This certification
or approval process can be viewed as the manufacturer making the case that the
system meets the criteria for certification or approval, and the third-party then
independently assessing the case to arrive at a decision. Assurance cases provide
a structure for making this case—using arguments supported by evidence to
justify a claim, typically in a hierarchical fashion. Generally, the top-level claim is
one about dependability properties of the system such as safety, trustworthiness

This work has been partially supported by NSF grants CNS-0931931 and CNS-
1035715

A. Ayoub—Currently employed at Mathworks.

© Springer International Publishing AG 2017
M. Huhn and L. Williams (Eds.): FHIES 2014/SEHC 2014, LNCS 9062, pp. 64–80, 2017.
DOI: 10.1007/978-3-319-63194-3_5

or reliability. An assurance case supports a claim *"x,"* such as *"the system is sufficiently safe"* or *"the system's software conforms to its requirements."*

Demonstrating such claims to the satisfaction of all concerned can be quite difficult. In stable and well-established fields such as avionics and medical devices, a prescriptive approach is commonly followed. A regulatory agency sets forth standards that must be followed (processes used during the development phase, tests that the system must pass, and so on), and the manufacturers must provide evidence showing that they followed the prescription [24]. Evidence collection to demonstrate adherence to prescribed standards is mandated by the prescription. However, parts of the argument linking the evidence produced during development to the ultimate claim being made about the system dependability are implicit. This could pose challenges to independent third-party assessors who have to fill in the missing pieces of the argument linking the supplied evidence to the claims. Assurance cases have attracted considerable interest and also have been adopted in domains where system safety is of particular concern.

The medical devices field, in particular, presents extra sources of challenges that must be considered due to the existence and nature of patients, who interact directly with the systems or become part of the system themselves. These patients are unpredictable unknowns. Additionally, the existence of patients affects how medical device companies approach their design and certification processes.

Depending on the goal of the assurance case, how it is structured and argued varies. In this survey, we focus on the safety assurance case. According to Bloomfield, a safety assurance case is a *"documented body of evidence that provides a convincing and valid argument that a system is adequately safe for a given application in a given environment"* [7]. The vendor provides a claim of safety and the evidence to sufficiently substantiate that claim. The case is then evaluated by a regulatory agency that must decide if the system(s) with that software can be used in the market. The responsibility to make the assurance case and demonstrate the safety of the system(s) using the software rests on the vendor instead of on the regulatory agency.

Confidence in the reasoning as well as in the evidence must be considered carefully when evaluating an assurance case. Grigorova and Maibaum introduce a working definition for confidence in an assurance case as *"the quality or state of being certain that the assurance case is appropriately and effectively structured, and correct"* [13]. This working definition applies to both the assurance case developers, who must have confidence in their case before the system is delivered, and the assurance case reviewers, such as a regulatory agency, who must develop adequate confidence in the case before they approve a system for use.

A necessary aspect of confidence is uncertainty; more uncertainty reduces confidence. Bloomfield suggests that the best way to indicate confidence and uncertainty is through the use of probability [7]. Higher uncertainty reduces the probability of the confidence. Since uncertainty is inherent in the world, when making assurance cases, uncertainty must be addressed, either implicitly or explicitly. Engineers and researchers have necessarily had to figure out how to deal with uncertainty in their various approaches to assurance cases. A possible approach is to classify uncertainty into two types—aleatory (statistical) or epistemic (systematic). Aleatory uncertainty relates to "the intrinsic randomness of a phenomenon" [19]. These uncertainties are the "known unknowns" and are quantified by probability distributions. Examples would be the overinfusion in an infusion pump or human error when calculating drug amounts. Another source of aleatory uncertainty that easily could be forgotten is residual ones - i.e., after a hazard has been deemed mitigated, there could be a small chance that it actually was not. Epistemic uncertainty is "presumed as being caused by a lack of knowledge (or data)," or the "unknown unknowns" [19]. Examples would include faults in logical reasoning that the reasoner was not even aware of, or a sequence of inputs that had not been anticipated in the development and design process. A goal for uncertainty researchers is to reduce epistemic uncertainty to aleatory so that it can be modeled. Recently, there has been more focus on quantifying epistemic uncertainty through methods such as Dempster-Shafer theory or Bayesian analysis [27].

Researchers approach confidence and uncertainty in assurance cases usually through one of two ways—a qualitative analysis or a quantitative one. The qualitative view to dealing with aleatory uncertainty is to remove it, such as by narrowing the world-view to such a point that there is still sufficient confidence in the assurance case but there are no more unknowns. The qualitative view to dealing with epistemic uncertainty is to reason it away. The quantitative approach to uncertainty generally uses the fact that uncertainty reduces confidence—if one has 70% confidence in an argument, then one has 30% uncertainty.

This paper surveys how researchers have reasoned about confidence and uncertainty, first by organizing their work into whether they took a qualitative or quantitative approach, then by analyzing the sources of uncertainty present in their approaches and if those are aleatory or epistemic. Lastly, the paper concludes with a summary and a discussion of directions for future exploration; there has not been one approach that is fully adequate for the current state of assurance cases. As such, we believe that further work is needed to develop an uncertainty reasoning framework drawing on the strengths of current approaches.

2   Reasoning About Confidence and Uncertainty

Bertolino and Strigini [4] looked into the difference between the two extreme approaches to reasoning about software faults, "statistical" (quantitative) and "perfectionist" (qualitative). We follow the same premise for the rest of this section, but with a focus on how the research groups have reasoned about uncertainty. First, the work is separated into qualitative or quantitative approaches to reasoning about uncertainty (not qualitative or quantitative approaches to reasoning about assurance cases). Then, the subsection is further subdivided into three sections: (1) a summary of the research methods used, with a focus on how they reasoned about confidence; (2) a discussion of how the research groups have reasoned about uncertainty and into what category the uncertainties fall; and (3) a discussion of our views on these works.

2.1   Qualitative: Logical Argumentation

The structure of the argument plays an important role in the confidence in the assurance case. Researchers have focused on correct, logical argumentation structures to clearly convey how the claim, in a given context, can be inferred from the evidence provided. Uncertainty may then be dealt with by checking over the argumentation as well as by narrowing the context.

Tim Kelly presented the idea of using "argumentation structure" for assurance cases [17]. He used safety arguments to get the safety evidence needed to meet safety requirements. He developed the idea further into a formalized argumentation structure called the Goal Structured Notation (GSN)—a symbol-based language intended to help formulate assurance cases.

R.D. Hawkins et al. introduced the idea of the "assured safety argument" by separating an assurance case into two parts—the safety assurance case and the confidence case [14]. Instead of looking for ways to assess confidence implicit in an assurance case, they suggest making the argument for confidence explicit by constructing a second case—the confidence case—for the safety assurance case. The main idea is that the assurance case and the associated justification for it are two separate entities and should be treated as such. Since confidence is central to assessment, leaving it implicit or intermixed in a one-part assurance case can be a major source of confusion both for the party making the assurance case (how to justify the confidence) and the party reviewing it (how to factor in the confidence). The assurance case developers mark the locations on the "assurance argument" where more justification is needed, and these are then addressed in the "confidence argument." The direct and specific connection points between the two cases help ensure that the confidence argument contains no extraneous information beyond what is necessary to strengthen the assurance argument.

Uncertainty Reasoning. Kelly and Rob Weaver view uncertainty in a qualitative way [18,29]. For epistemic uncertainty, if the argument made in the assurance claim is *sufficiently* well-structured, there should be no unknowns. If potential sources of epistemic uncertainty still exist, then one needs to go back into the assurance case and figure out which part needs to be better structured to remove uncertainty. Options to deal with aleatory uncertainty include resolving it, such as determining a way to eliminate it, or arguing that it does not impact the overall claim (at least not enough to change its credibility).

Kelly provides a "step-by-step" guide for assurance case reviewers where he points out inconsistencies for which reviewers should look, biases that might be inadvertently (or purposefully) inserted, and sources of weak or incorrect reasoning [18]. While not expressly stated as confidence or uncertainty, these two qualities exist innately for a reviewer when reviewing an assurance case. A developer can also introduce sources of epistemic uncertainty, thus unknowingly influencing evidence or arguments. Weak reasoning and biases, if caught by the reviewer, can reduce the confidence he or she may have in the case.

Hawkins also holds the view that the scope of the assurance case should be narrowed to the point that no aleatory uncertainty exists [15]. He defines safety assurance as *"[a] qualitative statement expressing the degree of confidence that a safety claim is true"* [15]. If the argument is believable or probable, and all of the uncertainties (whether aleatory or epistemic) are known (but cannot be neutralized for one reason or another), then there is still high confidence in the argument and one does not have to worry about the uncertainties. This "sufficient confidence" is established in the confidence argument part of the "assured safety argument" [14]. The confidence argument has multiple purposes—it has to establish sufficient overall confidence in the assurance case, it has to justify the corresponding parts of the assurance argument, and it has to address the uncertainties that exist in the assurance argument.

Discussion. If everything has been considered that possibly could be of interest in the "world," then, as Kelly, Weaver, Hawkins et al. suggest, there would be no uncertainty. Nevertheless, this is not realistic. Epistemic uncertainty always exists, especially when interacting with the real world. It is not feasible to account for every possible eventuality, simply because there will always be something that cannot be explained or anticipated. It makes good sense, however, to try: a reason why engineers must talk to domain experts to understand the world when building new products or improving old ones.

Hawkins' narrowing of the world view to eliminate aleatory uncertainty can be understood in a similar fashion. If one is building a new insulin pump, it would be reasonable to consider non-diabetic persons as outside the scope of the world, so the issue of, "What if a non-diabetic person used this machine?" would be eliminated with the solution, "That is outside the scope of the system under consideration". The risk here is that the narrowing of the scope may exclude situations or usage scenarios that may in actuality occur. For example, the extensive use of medical devices and pharmaceutics "off label" (used in situations for which approval has not been granted) could be excluded from an assurance case's scope to focus on a small and well understood patient population. This may, however, introduce uncertainty (both aleatory and epistemic) with respect to the reasonableness of this narrowing.

While the idea of separating the confidence case from the assurance argument achieves an important separation of concerns, since the assurance case itself has the propensity to grow rapidly and become increasingly complex (to create, check, and evaluate), the confidence argument is likely to be just as complex as the original assurance case. We suspect that, especially for safety-critical systems, dealing with uncertainties using qualitative approaches entails some inherent difficulties that cannot be completely eliminated by better assurance case structuring alone.

Unlike quantitative approaches, which attempt to represent confidence as a numeric value that might hide the nuances behind that number, the qualitative approach focuses on the reasoning and rationale behind any confidence value that could (some say arbitrarily) be placed in a confidence argument. Hawkins et al. point out that to arrive at a numerical value for assurance case confidence, one needs to go through the process of logical reasoning that is being used in their argument structures [14]. Therefore, one could view the quantitative approaches as requiring a foundation of qualitative analyses, without which numbers may be incorrectly adjusted to fit the end goal.

2.2   Qualitative: Baconian Probability

John Goodenough et al. approach confidence in assurance cases through *eliminative induction*—increasing confidence by removing sources of doubt and using Baconian probability to represent confidence [11]. First, they identify sources of doubt, called "defeaters"—that is, anything that could bring down confidence in the assurance case, and then work towards removing each source of doubt or proving that it is not relevant, ("eliminating" them). As more sources of doubt are eliminated, the confidence in the claim grows. A potential source of confusion with Baconian probability is that it must not be treated like actual probability. For instance, if there are 12 sources of doubt and 8 are eliminated, then $\frac{8}{12}$ sources of doubt are eliminated is the only valid conclusion, and we have $\frac{8}{12}$ confidence. This is to be considered as qualitatively different from $\frac{2}{3}$ as a confidence measure.

Uncertainty Reasoning. In this approach, sources of doubt are similar to sources of uncertainty. There is no specific separation between aleatory and epistemic—both can be sources of doubt. As doubts are identified and eliminated uncertainty decreases. Using the previous example, if 12 sources of doubt have been identified, and 8 sources have been eliminated, we still have $\frac{4}{12}$ (not the same as $\frac{1}{3}$) uncertainty in the assurance case. However, there is no way to remove all sources of doubt. They acknowledge that uncertainty will never be fully eliminated as it is not possible to find out all sources of doubt, recognizing, without naming, the existence of epistemic uncertainty.

Discussion. The use of eliminative induction and Baconian probability to deal with uncertainty in assurance cases is unique to the approach of Goodenough et al. Confidence is not the absence of doubt; it is showing the lack of basis for its presence. Thus, it depends on identifying the sources of doubts, which can be problematic for epistemic uncertainty. Further, eliminating a large number of identified doubts does not (or should not) necessarily proportionally increase confidence—presence of a large number of identified doubts may lead one to question if there are more—unidentified—ones. If simply eliminating more defeaters increases confidence, then one could add a large number of defeaters and eliminate them to artificially increase confidence. The authors acknowledge this issue, but argue that in reality there are only a finite number of those that are of consequence. In a way, they follow the world/scope-narrowing approach followed by the previous qualitative researchers.

Confidence values are accumulated over an assurance case by simply summing up the Baconian probabilities from the leaf nodes of the assurance argument structure. As an example, if we had a claim supported by three pieces of evidence, with confidence in the evidences at $\frac{9}{12}$, $\frac{2}{3}$, and $\frac{1}{2}$, then the overall confidence for the claim would be $\frac{12}{17}$. This approach is rather straightforward. However, this treats all defeaters as equally important, which may not be appropriate; as the authors acknowledge, some defeaters may need to have more weight than others in determining confidence.

An advantage of the Baconian approach over Pascalian approaches (Sect. 2.3) can be illustrated by an example provided by Goodenough et al. [11]. If some claim is based on four independent sub-claims, each with an associated confidence of 0.999, their (Pascalian) combination would result in a confidence of $0.999^4 = 0.996$ for the claim. If some evidence now establishes 3 out of those 4 sub-claims to be true (1 confidence), then the overall confidence increases to $1^3 \times 0.999 = 0.999$, not much of a growth. However, using Baconian probabilities, starting at $\frac{0}{4}$ overall confidence ("invalid sub-claim" as defeaters), the new evidence raises it to $\frac{3}{4}$, clearly highlighting the significance of the evidence.

2.3 Quantitative: Pascalian Probability

Assurance and confidence appear to be linked in the view of Robin Bloomfield et al. [7]. When reviewing assurance cases, there is always a bias, affected by how much the reviewer trusts what he or she is reviewing. While the qualitative researchers sought to lessen this bias by well structured arguments, Bloomfield et al. preferred to use probabilities. Since there is never certainty in the world, probabilities are the best way to show this uncertainty. Their work has brought forth the idea that multi-legged arguments can support each other and give higher confidence to a claim, and the idea that when one has a high degree of confidence that a system satisfies a high level safety assurance, one has an even higher degree of confidence that the same system satisfies a lower level of safety assurance. Bloomfield et al. also developed their own argumentation structure, called Claims, Arguments, and Evidence notation (CAE), to reason about assurance cases [6].

Bev Littlewood and David Wright believe that probability, especially Bayesian probability, is the best way to address confidence [22]. They use an idealized, reduced example to make a formal analysis of confidence using Bayesian Belief Networks. Specifically, they looked at whether two *diverse* legs of an argument would help increase the confidence in the assurance case and found the answer to be *yes*, most of the time.

Xingyu Zhao et al. categorically state that they believe the quantitative approach is better and aligned more closely with how humans think and reason [31]. To this end, they developed a framework to assess confidence in assurance cases. Starting with a structured argument meta-model (that supports GSN [17], CAE [6], and TRUST-IT [9]), they map the meta-model onto Toulmin's argumentation theory model [28]. This is converted to a Bayesian Belief Network (BBN) via four branches of reasoning – justified premises, adequate information, justified applicable warrant, and justified assumption that no exceptions apply. In the BBN, the leaf nodes are then set to prior probability values and the non-leaf nodes are assigned a conditional probability table whose numbers are from "field related statistical data" and "expert judgments" [31].

To John Rushby, an assurance case is composed of two components: communication and reasoning [25]. He argues that given enough parameters, it is possible to strive for the "possibly perfect" piece of software [24]. One can look towards a value for the "probability of perfection," which can then be related to confidence. He later argues, similar to Hawkins et al. [15], that if one narrows the scope enough to what is relevant, then perfection is possible as all uncertainties would have been eliminated. He approaches assurance cases and confidence recursively, building up confidence from the leaf nodes (*"substantiated claims about a subsystem can be used as evidence in a parent case"*).

Uncertainty Reasoning. Bloomfield et al. say that we use probability *because* there is uncertainty. In their view, uncertainty surely exists in the environment, and it is best shown by using probabilities for confidence values [7]. Here, uncertainty is the complement of confidence in an assurance case—e.g., 0.8 confidence means 0.2 uncertainty.

Peter Bishop et al. address the issue of epistemic uncertainty in reliability cases as it relates specifically to the probability of failure on demand [5]. Uncertainty always exists, especially epistemic uncertainty, and it needs to be dealt with when developing assurance cases. Their approach is to suggest the use of Bayesian Networks, relating back to Bloomfield et al.'s initial suggestion of probability.

Littlewood and Wright's use of Bayesian Belief Networks indicate their recognition of epistemic uncertainty [22]. To them, confidence's complement is doubt, which they model with probabilities in a BBN. Their results from looking more into multi-legged arguments for assurance cases show that depending on the nature of the extra "legs" in the argument, these legs can increase or reduce confidence in the original claim, a fact which is not wholly intuitive.

The use of Bayesian Belief Networks by Zhao et al. point to a desire to quantify the epistemic uncertainty that exists in assurance cases [31]. The use of prior probability values is the result of reducing epistemic uncertainty to aleatory uncertainty for the leaf nodes, to be propagated back through the BBN.

Rushby asserts that there will always be unknowns [24]. He believes that we should formalize the assurance case review process as much as possible to reduce the amount of information that needs "human review." There is a notional perfect system, which is impossible to achieve, and so one should build towards that perfect system. Software is reliable and has predictable behavior, but its environment, riddled with epistemic doubt, is not [25]. He maintains that reasoning is a logical process which can be mechanized, while communication, involving human factors, is epistemic in nature. In Rushby's world, if the software never fails, we have reached perfection—a probability of one. He argues that the more verification and validation that has been done on a piece of software, the greater the "probability of being perfect." He views verification as part of the logical reasoning, which is reducible and can hopefully be formalized, and validation as dealing with epistemic doubt. The goal then is to reduce the epistemic doubt to the point where logical analysis can take over. Then, only the leaf nodes have epistemic uncertainty and once these are addressed the rest of the model can be formally analyzed.

Discussion. Bloomfield et al., along with Littlewood and Wright, say that multi-legged arguments can provide more confidence for a claim. Littlewood and Wright formally show this with a reduced example; they also show that confidence may be reduced by a seemingly supportive second leg argument. This issue is looked into further by in Sect. 2.6 – Ayoub et al. explore ways that evidence can combine to support or detract from the claim [2].

While probabilities help quantify confidence, using a single number ignores the subtle nuances in reasoning about uncertainty. The use of probability is a logical approach to quantifying confidence and uncertainty, but might be too coarse of an approach. More recent works address this issue specifically when addressing epistemic uncertainty, such as the one by Bloomfield et al. [5].

Zhao et al. develop a framework and they show several interesting results, but the specifics of the process employed are not clear from their work [31]. They provide simple guidelines and advocate using "common sense" to quantify uncertainty, but details seem to be lacking.

Rushby directly addresses the idea of "epistemic doubt", but does not view it in the same way we have approached it here [25]. In contrast to our categorization of uncertainty into epistemic and aleatory, he focuses on logic and doubt. As such, aleatory uncertainty is not specifically mentioned. He views the reasoning behind the connections between arguments as where there is no uncertainty (it is logic), while we argue that this is perhaps where much of the epistemic uncertainty exists.

2.4   Quantitative: The Confidence Toolkit

Lukasz Cyra and Janusz Górski also developed their own argument structure and notation, similar to Kelly's GSN [17] or Bloomfield's CAE [6], called Trust-IT [9]. Where they differ from Kelly is the view that a sufficiently detailed, complete assurance case requires so much information that these argument structures become huge, unwieldy and difficult to navigate. The size makes reviewing the assurance case especially difficult. Their solution is to look at the language used in "expert assessments" and quantify it.

First, they generate a confidence versus decision plot. One axis is the "decision scale," which has four possible values representing decisions that could be made by the reviewer—rejectable, opposable (a soft reject), tolerable (a soft accept), or acceptable. The other axis is the "confidence scale," which has six possible values ranging from absolute "lack of confidence" to total "for sure" confidence. This is all plotted on a single two dimensional graph. When one has high confidence and acceptability, that is for sure a go (accept). When one has high confidence and opposability, then that indicates a stop (reject).

They next map this rectangular "assessment scale" onto a decision triangle – Josang's opinion triangle [16]. The "accept" and "reject" corners of the rectangle map onto the base of the triangle, and all decision points that correspond to "lack of confidence" map to a single point of uncertainty at the apex of the triangle. They conclude that when one has high confidence and an acceptable decision, there is a strong belief in the acceptability of the assurance case. Likewise, when there is high confidence and a rejectable decision, there is a strong disbelief in the acceptability of the assurance case. But when there is high uncertainty, no decision can be made. They effectively move from a two choice scale (accept or reject) to a three-choice scale (accept, reject, wait). The NOR-STA tool created by them provides a visual breakdown of a trust case, a decision, and the confidence/uncertainty in that decision and presents the decision scale on a user-friendly graphical interface. It provides a summary from the aggregation of expert assessors' opinions, along with a value for the uncertainty resulting from the aggregation. The intent is present all information to the final decision maker.

Uncertainty Reasoning. Cyra and Górski view uncertainty as lack of confidence and equate high levels of uncertainty with inability to make a decision [9]. A strong lack of confidence represents extreme uncertainty. Something that has been assessed as "with very low confidence opposable" is weak on multiple points. It is not a strong reject or accept on the decision scale, but it also has a fairly high level of uncertainty, casting doubt onto any decision that could be made. By mapping this graph onto Josang's triangle, the authors highlight the importance of uncertainty. Everything is in doubt when uncertainty dominates as it clouds the decision making process. They present a third option beyond "accept" or "reject", namely "wait" – wait for more information, until the uncertainty is removed and the confidence increased.

In the NOR-STA tool, the confidence in the assurance case is presented to the reviewer on a slider scale, while the uncertainty is shown on Josang's Triangle, so that with one quick glance, the reviewer can see clearly the confidence and the uncertainty associated with that confidence. The uncertainty represented is epistemic in nature, as it deals with the communication from the reviewers. Aleatory uncertainty may be taken into consideration by the reviewers in formulating their assessment but is not explicitly dealt with in the NOR-STA tool.

Discussion. Like Bloomfield et al., Cyra and Górski appear to view uncertainty as directly related to confidence. Additionally, they look at trust, represented by the belief or disbelief in the claim, which is wholly separate from confidence and uncertainty. Their use of the opinion triangle shows their approach to reasoning about uncertainty. It follows that when one has a lack of confidence, there is uncertainty. Therefore, one cannot make a decision when there is high uncertainty. Whereas one might look at Bloomfield et al.'s view as high uncertainty implies low confidence and thus a rejection, Cyra's approach is that a firm reject only applies when one has high confidence in the rejection. What they do not talk about is what to do when there are high levels of uncertainty. We believe it means that more information is needed, and no sound decision can be made until that uncertainty has been reduced or eliminated.

Their work also seeks to quantify language, which has a lot of subjectivity ("tolerable" versus "acceptable," for instance). Very few others, such as Lorenzo

Stringini [26], have attempted to do something similar. However, human communication typically involves such subjective terms from which an objective decision must be derived. It is therefore useful to explore this deeper and the area holds potential for further study.

2.5   Quantitative: Multi-component

Current popular assurance case tools such as GSN, CAE, or NOR-STA can very quickly and very easily balloon to such an extent that they are no longer beneficial to or navigable by the reviewer. In fact, too much information can obscure the argument or even be used to hide flaws. One quantitative approach by researchers is through the use of multi-component assurance cases. By separating the assurance case into multiple parts, the hope is that overall complexity is reduced while clarity of the arguments is increased.

Ewen Denney et al. continue Hawkins et al.'s work on a separate confidence case, but with a quantitative approach through the use of Bayesian Belief Networks [10]. This work represents an acknowledgement that numbers, when used prudently, can be helpful in reasoning about assurance cases. Their basic premise starts from a safety argument created using GSN. Then, following Hawkins et al., they create a confidence argument. Lastly, the nodes are quantified.

John Knight also embraced the idea of partitioning assurance cases, specifically, by separating the arguments into three different types—design, confidence, and operational [20]. Design arguments are used for a "desired safety property," confidence arguments deal with acceptability or believability of the components of assurance case, while operational arguments argue that assumptions made in the design argument will be true in an operational context.

Marc Bender et al. address confidence as one step in a multi-component software certification process [3]. They have split the process of certification into different categories of required information: evidence, confidence, determination, and certification. Similar to Knight, they address separation of concerns - when talking about evidence, and bringing about pieces of it as part of certification, one should only be concerned with the evidence, and *not* such qualities as trustworthiness, confidence, etc. When dealing with confidence, one only concerns oneself with aspects that relate directly to that. Evaluating evidence increases confidence, and this stops when one has reached the necessary satisfaction level. In their work, assurance cases are used as a representation of confidence. Just like how certification was broken down into four elements, confidence is also broken down into three necessary components: veracity about sources (trustworthiness), validity (soundness), and adequacy (sufficiency of knowledge).

Grigorova and Maibaum explore the analogy between confidence in assurance cases and the weight of evidence in law [13]. Looking at current assurance case confidence and their flaws in reasoning, the authors want to establish an exhaustive and complete compendium of relevant knowledge, one "living document" for each domain so that both developers and reviewers can see a baseline of what must be included. They start with a working definition of confidence that was introduced at the beginning of this paper, and stress that their goal is to achieve safety, not to satisfy a bunch of check boxes (focus on the process, not the end product), hence the suggestion for the compendium of evidence. Essentially, they are expanding upon Bender et al.'s multi-component approach by separating the *weight* of the evidence from other factors that may influence confidence.

Uncertainty Reasoning. Denney et al.'s use of BBNs show their recognition of the existence of epistemic uncertainty in their confidence arguments, as BBNs are generally considered the best way to treat epistemic uncertainty [27].

Bender et al. are of the viewpoint that uncertainty leads directly to a decrease in confidence [3]. They quantify the aleatory uncertainty by using random variables (usually normally distributed) with the means and variances affected by prior beliefs or parent nodes. Epistemic uncertainty is dealt with when a joint distribution is then computed on these random variables, and everything is tied together via a Bayesian Belief Network. They use the BBN to calculate confidence in the safety argument.

Greenwell et al. looked at fallacies made in system safety arguments [12]. As stated earlier, we believe that flaws in reasoning are sources of epistemic uncertainty, as there are multiple causes of such reasoning errors and, as demonstrated by Greenwell et al., such errors are difficult even for experts to correctly recognize and identify.

Rodes et al. equate confidence to belief in their work [23]. They create a generic framework for measuring a property (they use security but state that it can also be used for other areas, such as safety) via confidence. This confidence is directly related to belief, and can be reduced by doubt, which is caused by uncertainty. They discuss sources of doubt in assurance cases that include incorrect inferences, faulty evidence, or inaccurate goals. These are all sources of epistemic uncertainty.

Grigorova and Maibaum view uncertainty as the opposite of confidence [13]. They understand that it has a role in reducing confidence, and the use of weighted evidence would also impact uncertainty in different ways. By seeking to create a complete compendium of evidence, they attempt to turn epistemic uncertainty to aleatory, and ultimately eliminate some uncertainties.

Discussion. One issue with multi-component assurance cases is that while seeking to avoid the complications associated with complex and huge assurance cases, we possibly end up overloading reviewers with even more information, just presented differently. Instead of one complicated assurance case, the fear is that we now have three or four equally complicated assurance cases.

Denney et al. address a weakness in their approach when talking about evidence weights [10]. Like Goodenough et al. [11], the authors do not provide for a solution if some components of the argument are more important than others. Their assumption is the weights are equal. As seen earlier, Grigorova and Maibaum also looked into weighted evidence, as will Ayoub et al. [1]. Cyra and Górski's NOR-STA tool allows assessors to assign weights to premises of certain warrants [9].

An issue in Grigorova and Maibuam's work is that they do not seem to be addressing directly who should bear this burden of considering evidence weights [13]. The authors do go back and forth a bit on this issue. Should it be the assurance case developer who makes sure all the evidence is accounted for or the reviewer who has to check that the evidence has all been included?

2.6 Quantitative: Confirmation Bias and Weighted Evidence

Anaheed Ayoub et al. start with the idea of confirmation bias, as noted by Leveson [21], which almost always exists when dealing with human judgment [1]. The basic premise is that we all have our preconceived notions, and these preconceptions influence our decisions and how we think in subtle, sometimes unrecognized ways. We are more likely to believe something if it aligns with what we have previously believed. So people who are structuring the assurance case might (possibly unintentionally) bias the evidence they use towards the claim and minimize evidence that might weaken it. Leveson further suggests that one way to combat confirmation bias when arguing that a system is safe is to use a counter-argument [21]. An example would be, instead of trying to argue that a system is safe, have the manufacturer argue that the system is unsafe. Then they are forced to consider evidence that previously would have been rejected.

Ayoub et al. take this idea in a different way, by focusing on the reviewers and having them argue for the sufficiency and the insufficiency of an argument [1]. The question they ask is, *"are the premises of the argument 'strong enough' to support the conclusions being drawn?"* The authors ask reviewers to assess a claim's sufficiency and insufficiency, forcing them to look at the why of what they think. Then, the difference from one of these two arguments is viewed as the uncertainty. For instance, given a claim "the device is safe to use," a reviewer evaluates its sufficiency at 80%, or 0.8. For the same claim, the reviewer is asked to evaluate its insufficiency (or, thought of differently, the reviewer is asked to evaluate the claim "the device is NOT safe to use"). He or she evaluates this at 10%, or 0.1. This means there is another 10% of the reviewer's opinion that is not accounted for - this is the uncertainty. By asking the reviewer to evaluate the insufficiency of the claim, Ayoub et al. seek to avoid confirmation bias.

Ayoub et al. also sought to create "a systematic approach to justifying confidence" in safety arguments [2]. Just as Weaver et al. sought to create a systematic approach to evaluating safety arguments [29], Ayoub et al. now apply similar ideas to the confidence arguments as introduced by Hawkins et al. [14]. The authors encourage a prescriptive approach (using what they call a "common characteristics map") to identifying the system hazards and deficits in the assurance case, mitigating these defects, then putting it all together in the confidence case. This all starts with the idea of masses and weights.

Uncertainty Reasoning. Ayoub et al. use masses and weights as representations of confidence in [2]. Higher confidence means a higher mass, implying a better or stronger argument. Arguments and evidences are weighted depending on their strengths. As part of their approach, they separated the evidence that the reviewers are examining into four types: alternate, disjoint, overlap, and containment, based partially on Dempster-Shafer theory. When the mass is zero, full uncertainty is implied. Such a missing mass, when used in a formula to calculate the overall sufficiency of an argument, can affect the total mass (and thus the total confidence), depending on the weight of the missing mass. The use of Dempster-Shafer theory implies that the authors acknowledge the existence of epistemic uncertainty. Aleatory uncertainties affect the mass of the evidence.

Discussion. This intriguing approach needs further development and refinement. It is counter-intuitive for some people to think about arguing for insufficiency, and it is not easy for most people to argue against themselves. It is even more counter-intuitive to think about all of the confidences adding up to one. One wonders if it is possible for a reviewer to give his or her sufficiency an 80% confidence and his or her insufficiency a 50% confidence. Where would the uncertainty be then? We argue that this should be allowed, and the excess 30% confidence over 100% would represent the uncertainty. There are a lot of limitations that the authors themselves admit.

While previous researchers mentioned the importance of weighting evidence, Ayoub et al. are the only group to actually consider it thus far, and they provide a logical solution. They also look further into how different pieces of evidence can combine to either increase or reduce confidence, in a similar fashion to how other researchers looked at multi-legged arguments.

3 Conclusions

We have briefly surveyed recent work on safety assurance cases and their potential usefulness in safety critical systems. A key issue that plagues assurance cases is uncertainty, which necessarily exists in the real world. Uncertainly can be categorized as aleatory or epistemic. Researchers have used a variety of methods to handle uncertainty inherent in assurance arguments supporting system dependability claims. We have attempted to categorize the uncertainty addressed by various methods, which is somewhat complicated by additional factors – the model used and the situation in which the method is applied play a role.

Qualitative approaches usually try to narrow the scope of the assurance case world to such a point that all uncertainties have been either eliminated or shown to be inconsequential. Quantitative approaches acknowledge that uncertainty always exists and must be dealt with, usually through its impact on confidence values. Since aleatory and epistemic uncertainty vary in how they are treated quantitatively, a clear distinction is crucial.

In our view, there has not been one approach that is fully adequate for the current state of assurance cases, though many approaches have novel ideas that address important considerations. It is our belief that to comprehensively handle uncertainty, one may need to employ a combination of approaches, perhaps including new techniques that have yet to be developed. While we do not yet have such a solution, we think it must have some essential ingredients.

Weighting evidence enables a more accurate reflection of the real world, and as such, is a minimum necessity in assurance cases. If we can get to a point in an assurance case where the leaf nodes only contain aleatory uncertainty, and epistemic uncertainty only exists in the other nodes, then perhaps it would be feasible to apply formal reasoning methods to the argumentation between the leaf and non-leaf nodes.

We believe that probability should be used to quantify uncertainty, especially if any sort of mechanization process is desired. How weighted evidence ties into Bayesian Belief Networks is an area ripe for exploring.

Another issue that must be addressed is the lack of consistency in the terminology and working definitions used by different researchers, which makes comparison techniques and combining approaches challenging. While this is to be expected in a new area, we believe the field is now maturing to the point where a common foundation would better serve further study.

A third issue is how little research has focused on the human factors, with some giving up before even starting, and others trying to minimize this as much as possible so as to avoid dealing with it. As this is an aspect that is unavoidable, it is worth a deeper look. A fourth issue is that uncertainty is a vast research area in its own right. Before dwelling deeply into reasoning about uncertainty in assurance cases, it would serve well to understand the foundational principles in reasoning about uncertainty in general. Lastly, the importance of proper assurance case technique must be underscored. It is far too easy for assurance case creators to go overboard and put too much and unnecessary information in an assurance case, potentially losing the argument that is being made or obscuring shortcomings that might exist in the evidence. Assurance cases should have clear, convincing, and preferably concise arguments.

While we have presented a survey of approaches to reasoning about confidence and uncertainty in assurance cases, an obvious question would be which method is superior? To answer this question requires a comparative evaluation between techniques. While we feel that this is beyond the scope of the original intentions of this work, we would like to present some thoughts on this issue.

Context is of utmost importance when choosing the best method to analyze confidence and uncertainty in assurance cases. The source of the uncertainty will also have an impact on the method used to address it. As we have shown, there are a variety of methods to convey, analyze, and evaluate confidence and uncertainty. At times, one method might prove to be more informative than others, while this same method might be insufficient in other situations.

For infusion pumps in the United States which expect to undergo FDA regulation, which require assurance cases as part of the approval process, exact confidence and uncertainty values might be less important as the overall reasoning [8]. As such, a qualitative approach might be reasonable. The purpose of the assurance case is for the manufacturer to show that they have reasoned about their device, similar to the logical reasoning as espoused by Kelly, Hawkins, Weaver, et al.

In the UK, the Healthy and Safety at Work Act uses the phrase "so far as is reasonably practicable" - which is a qualitative goal [30]. As such, while it is possible to use a quantitative analysis and then map it onto a qualitative scale, one could reasonably use logical argumentation to show that the goal has been achieved without the use of any specific quantifiers.

On the other hand, a manufacturer that is attempting to show that their system is an improvement over another might benefit more from a quantitative approach. If more confidence or less uncertainty was demonstrated, quantitatively.

References

1. Ayoub, A., Chang, J., Sokolsky, O., Lee, I.: Assessing the overall sufficiency of safety arguments. In: Safety-Critical Systems Club (2013)
2. Ayoub, A., Kim, B.G., Lee, I., Sokolsky, O.: A systematic approach to justifying sufficient confidence in software safety arguments. In: Ortmeier, F., Daniel, P. (eds.) SAFECOMP 2012. LNCS, vol. 7612, pp. 305–316. Springer, Heidelberg (2012). doi:10.1007/978-3-642-33678-2_26
3. Bender, M., Maibaum, T., Lawford, M., Wassyng, A.: Positioning verification in the context of software/system certification. In: Proceedings of the 11th International Workshop on Automated Verification of Critical Systems (2011)
4. Bertolino, A., Strigini, L.: Assessing the risk due to software faults: estimates of failure rate versus evidence of perfection. Softw. Testing Verification Reliab. 8(3), 155–166 (1998)
5. Bishop, P., Bloomfield, R., Littlewood, B., Povyakalo, A., Wright, D.: Towards a formalism for conservative claims about the dependability of software-based systems. IEEE Trans. Softw. Eng. 37(5), 708–717 (2011)
6. Bloomfield, R., Bishop, P.: Safety and assurance cases: past, present, and possible future - an adelard perspective. In: Making Systems Safe (2010)
7. Bloomfield, R.E., Littlewood, B., Wright, D.: Confidence: its role in dependability cases for risk assessment. In: International Conference on Dependable Systems and Networks (2007)
8. Chapman, R.: Safety assurance for embedded software in infusion pumps. In: Presented as a Keynote Talk at FHIES/SEHC (2014)
9. Cyra, L., Górski, J.: Supporting expert assessment of argument structures in trust cases. In: 9th International Probability Safety Assessment and Management Conference PSAM (2008)
10. Denney, E., Pai, G., Habli, I.: Towards measurement of confidence in safety cases. In: 2011 International Symposium on Empirical Software Engineering and Measurement (2011)
11. Goodenough, J.B., Weinstock, C.B., Klein, A.Z.: Toward a theory of assurance case confidence. Technical report, Carnegie Mellon (2012)
12. Greenwell, W.S., Knight, J.C., Holloway, C.M., Pease, J.J.: A taxonomy of fallacies in system safety arguments. In: International System Safety Conference (2006)
13. Grigorova, S., Maibaum, T.S.E.: Taking a page from the law books: considering evidence weight in evaluating assurance case confidence. In: Software Reliability Engineering Workshops (2013)
14. Hawkins, R.D., Kelly, T., Knight, J., Graydon, P.: A new approach to creating clear safety arguments. In: Advances in Systems Safety (2011)

15. Hawkins, R.D., Kelly, T.P.: Software safety assurance - what is sufficient? In: 4th IET International Conference on Systems Safety (2009)
16. Jøsang, A., Grandison, T.: Conditional inference in subjective logic. In: Proceedings of the 6th International Conference on Information Fusion (2003)
17. Kelly, T.: Arguing safety-a systematic approach to safety case management. PhD thesis, The University of York (1998)
18. Kelly, T.: Reviewing assurance arguments - a step-by-step approach. In: Safety Management Requirements for Defence System (2007)
19. Der Kiureghian, A., Ditlevsen, O.: Aleatory or epistemic? does it matter? J. Struct. Safety **31**(2), 105–112 (2008)
20. Knight, J.: Private e-mail communication (2014)
21. Leveson, N.: Cost-effective safety certification of software-intensive systems. In: Seventh Software Certification Consortium (2011)
22. Littlewood, B., Wright, D.: The use of multilegged arguments of increase confdience in safety claims for software-based sytems: a study based on a BBN analysis of an idealized example. IEEE Trans. Software Eng. **33**(5), 347–365 (2007)
23. Rodes, B.D., Knight, J.C., Wasson, K.S.: A security metric based on security arguments. In: WETSoM 2014 (2014)
24. Rushby, J.: Formalism in safety cases. In: Dale, C., Anderson, T. (eds.) Making Systems Safer, pp. 3–17. Springer, London (2010)
25. Rushby, J.: Logic and epistemology in safety cases. In: Proceedings of SafeComp, p. 32 (2013)
26. Strigini, L.: Engineering judgement in reliability and safety and its limits: what can we learn from research in psychology. Technical report, Centre for Software Reliability Technical report (1996)
27. Swiler, L.P., Paez, T.L., Mayes, R.L.: Epistemic uncertainty quantification tutorial. In: Proceedings of the IMAC-XXVII (2009)
28. Toulmin, S.: The Uses of Argument. Cambridge University Press, Cambridge (1958)
29. Weaver, R., Fenn, J., Kelly, T.: A pragmatic approach to reasoning about the assurance of safety arguments. In: 8th Australian Workshop on Safety Critical Systems and Software (SCS 2003) (2003)
30. Wilkinson, P.: The use of safety cases in certification and regulation by Nancy Leveson a review by Peter Wilkinson. Technical report, US Chemical Safety Board (2014)
31. Zhao, X., Zhang, D., Lu, M., Zeng, F.: A new approach to assessment of confidence in assurance cases. In: Ortmeier, F., Daniel, P. (eds.) SAFECOMP 2012. LNCS, vol. 7613, pp. 79–91. Springer, Heidelberg (2012). doi:10.1007/978-3-642-33675-1_7

Building Semantic Causal Models to Predict Treatment Adherence for Tuberculosis Patients in Sub-Saharan Africa

Olukunle A. Ogundele[1]([⊠]), Deshendran Moodley[3]([⊠]),
Christopher J. Seebregts[1,2]([⊠]), and Anban W. Pillay[1]([⊠])

[1] UKZN/CSIR Meraka Centre for Artificial Intelligence Research
and Health Architecture Laboratory, School of Mathematics,
Statistics and Computer Science,
University of KwaZulu-Natal, Durban, South Africa
zinmanship@yahoo.co.uk, chris@jembi.org,
Pillayw4@ukzn.ac.za
[2] Jembi Health Systems NPC, Cape Town, Durban, South Africa
[3] Department of Computer Science,
UCT/CSIR Meraka Centre for Artificial Intelligence Research,
University of Cape Town, Cape Town, South Africa
deshen@cs.uct.ac.za

Abstract. Poor adherence to prescribed treatment is a major factor contributing to tuberculosis patients developing drug resistance and failing treatment. Treatment adherence behaviour is influenced by diverse personal, cultural and socio-economic factors that vary between regions and communities. Decision network models can potentially be used to predict treatment adherence behaviour. However, determining the network structure (identifying the factors and their causal relations) and the conditional probabilities is a challenging task. To resolve the former we developed an ontology supported by current scientific literature to categorise and clarify the similarity and granularity of factors.

Keywords: Ontology · Decision network · Tuberculosis treatment adherence · Tuberculosis treatment failure

1 Introduction

Tuberculosis (TB) treatment failure is a significant challenge facing TB control programmes in sub-Saharan African countries resulting in increased rates of drug resistance, morbidity and mortality [1, 2]. Poor treatment adherence is an important predictor of TB treatment failure [3]. Treatment adherence is defined as the extent to which a patient adheres to an appropriate treatment guideline that includes medicine adherence behaviour, following a prescribed diet, and/or executing lifestyle changes [4]. Refusal or inability to follow a prescribed treatment guideline is termed non-adherence [5].

The importance of treatment adherence behaviour has prompted public health researchers to call for the transformation of intervention programmes, by introducing a more patient centred approach to complement the current programmatic approach of

© Springer International Publishing AG 2017
M. Huhn and L. Williams (Eds.): FHIES 2014/SEHC 2014, LNCS 9062, pp. 81–95, 2017.
DOI: 10.1007/978-3-319-63194-3_6

many treatment programs [4]. Patient-centred approaches include an understanding of existing behaviour and perceptions of target groups [4], how patient behaviour affects treatment compliance and how the social characteristics of patients affect their response to treatment [6]. TB treatment adherence behaviour (TAB) is a complex social phenomenon [3] with no general agreement on the similarity, granularity and the degree of influence of different factors [4, 3]. In addition, the diverse personal, cultural and socio-economic factors vary between countries, communities and social groups [3]. It is therefore challenging to identify distinguishing characteristics of potential treatment defaulters [4] in specific communities.

A decision network (DN) is a potentially useful modelling paradigm to model the complex factors and relationships that influence TAB. DN models are based on Bayesian networks (BN) which are used to represent vague and probabilistic causal relations between different variables [7, 8]. A DN can potentially be used to predict TAB and may be used as the basis for decision support tools to help TB programme coordinators identify and/or predict potential treatment default behaviour. Developing such networks for TAB requires significant modelling effort, including the identification of influencing factors, formalizing these factors to form the network's structure, determination of the weighting for the conditional probabilities, and consolidating evidence for learning the network. Expert knowledge and primary data sources are also required, particularly when dealing with unstructured data [9].

Ontologies can be useful to consolidate and represent categorical knowledge from an unstructured source of data. An ontology has been defined as an explicit specification of a conceptualization [10] and is a method that has already been used successfully to represent common knowledge in the public health domain [11, 12]. Ontologies have significant capability for structuring and classifying concepts and providing connections and relationships between concepts in an application domain [13].

This study describes an ontology for representing, consolidating and structuring the factors influencing the adherence behaviour of TB patients. The ontology categorises the factors and represents their effect on adherence behaviour and, crucially, enables the linking of factors to clinical studies that provide evidence for their predictive value. Furthermore, we show how the ontology can be used to construct a decision network model for particular TB communities.

The rest of the paper is structured as follows: Sect. 2 outlines previous work, Sect. 3 presents the ontology while Sect. 4 demonstrates its use in constructing decision networks. Section 5 concludes with a summary and pointers for future work.

2 Previous Work

Mathematical models have been used previously to model adherence behaviour. A machine-learning method was used to identify predictors for treatment adherence for heart failure patients [14]. A support vector machine was used for classification and analysis of the data collected directly from the patients. The study identified, among others, gender, age, education, and monthly income as predictors for medication adherence. The study stopped short of predicting medication adherence in heart failure patients and instead identified and analysed the variables that could affect medication adherence. The investigators were not able to draw any inferences with respect to the causal relationship between these predictors.

A cost-benefit mathematical modelling approach was used for describing treatment adherence for diabetic patients [15]. A synthesis of several psychological theories of medication compliance was used to produce a model that was tested using diabetic treatment adherence cases. The test was carried out at both population and individual levels, and it proved that a detailed "mechanistic" mathematical representation of medication adherence is possible and useful for the public health domain. This study however did not consider the structuring of the factors and did not draw any causal relationships between them.

A Bayesian network was used to identify and analyse non-compliance in glaucoma patients and to examine factors that motivate their poor adherence [16]. A model was developed to identify poor compliers by discriminating between low-compliance and moderate- or high-compliance patients.

Ontologies have been used to represent common knowledge in the bio-medical and public health domains. This includes disease representation and epidemiology [17, 11], heterogeneous information and system integration [12, 18], bio-medical information structuring [19, 20], and healthcare service support [21, 22]. An ontology was developed to model TB care pathways to help clinical officers access and retrieve the best available evidence from underlying medical databases [21]. An ontology was also used to classify the terminology used to describe standard laboratory test codes using TB as a case study [20]. A generic and extensible framework that can be used to assess patient adherence and persistence rates from production EMR data was developed in [23]. The framework used an ontology to represent different drugs and patient classification information.

3 An Ontology for Factors Influencing Adherence Behaviour

3.1 Categorising TB Treatment Adherence Influencing Factors

An ontology to categorize and represent the factors that influence treatment adherence behaviour of TB patients was developed. An extensive survey of the literature was first undertaken to compile a comprehensive list of factors affecting TAB in sub-Saharan Africa. Three qualitative review papers and fourteen case-based papers that dealt with the categorisation and consolidation of TAB casual factors were reviewed and provided background knowledge of the factors and their categories. The qualitative review papers provided common aspects of factors classification, while the other papers identified the various factors that influence TAB in sub-Saharan African countries.

The classifications presented in the review papers were done in order to better understand the factors [3, 24] and for proposing interventions [4]. This reveals earlier attempts to consolidate and categorise the factors to support intervention and decision-making in TB control. These papers presented similar models for the categories, but the description of the categories and the identified factors vary. The major categories identified across the three papers are: personal/patient-centred, clinical/therapy, health-care system, structural/economic, disease factor, social, health service, and condition related factors. The three papers reviewed include most of the categories with particular focus on factors that are peculiar to sub-Saharan Africa.

3.2   Ontology Development

The ontology was developed in the Ontology Web Language (OWL) using the Protégé tool[1]. The ontology categorises the factors, their effects on TAB and supporting evidence for the inclusion of the factor. The main classes in the ontology are the `InfluencingFactor` and `Evidence` classes. These classes have subclasses and are linked by object properties that define their relationships (see Figs. 1 and 2 below).

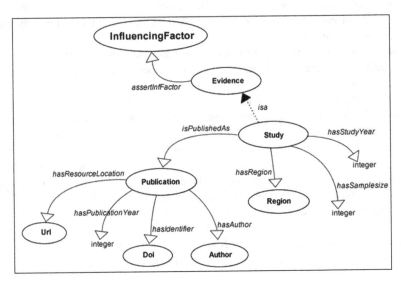

Fig. 1. Key concepts of the influencing factors ontology

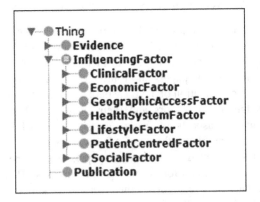

Fig. 2. High level classes of the ontology

---

[1] http://protege.stanford.edu/.

Influencing Factors Ontology: Classes Description

The Influencing Factor Class: InfluencingFactor

A factor is a characteristic or a group of characteristics of a TB patient that has been identified as influencing treatment adherence and is informed by research studies performed on one or more communities. To create the ontology, categories from the literature were refactored into seven comprehensive and unique categories to eliminate conceptual overlaps.

We identified unique factor categories from the literature that can be distinctly represented in the ontology. These are the patient centred, clinical, economic, social, health system, geographical access, and lifestyle related categories. Figure 2 shows these categories in Protégé. The ontology presently contains twenty-eight unique factors that are commonly identified as predictors of TAB in sub-Saharan Africa.

A hierarchical structure was used to represent the factors in the ontology. This made it possible to represent granularities of the factors. Figure 3 below shows the structure for the patient centred category as an example of the structure representing the InfluencingFactor class in the ontology.

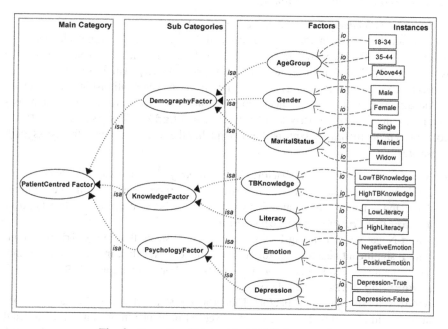

Fig. 3. Example of hierarchical CCF class ontology

The Evidence Class: Evidence

Evidence is formal or informal knowledge that provides supporting information for a TB patient's characteristic or group of characteristics as having influence on TAB. Evidence includes expert knowledge from review papers and scientific studies carried out on TB patients.

The Study Class: `Study`

This is a type of `Evidence` that is (an empirical) scientific study/research carried out in a region on some population (sample of patients) in a particular year or period. A `Study` is described with sets of attributes, which include the year of the study, the study region, and information about the scientific publication that reports the findings of the study. The `Study` class is defined as a sub-type of the `Evidence` class.

The Publication Class: `Publication`

A `Publication` represents any published document that is produced from a study. It has attributes such as the name of the author(s), year of publication, URL of the online location of the document, the digital object identifier (doi) for the document.

The Region Class: `Region`

A `Region` refers to the place where the study was carried out (study location), it may be the town, city, province or country of the study. The `Region` class is related to the `Study` class and is limited to countries in this paper. It will be expanded, in future work, into a spatial ontology, using the "`partOf`" relation to connectspatial entities (city, district, province, country).

Class Relationships in the Ontology

Evidence → Influencing-factor: `assertInfFactor`

The relationship between the `Evidence` and `InfluencingFactor` classes is an assertion. A TAB influencing factor is asserted by some evidence or some evidence asserts some TAB influencing factors. For example, a `Study`, which is an `Evidence`, asserts that `Male` gender is an `InfluencingFactor`. The relationship is represented by the `assertInfFactor` object property, an abbreviation for assert-influencing-factor with the inverse property `infFactorAssertedBy`. The `assertInfFactor` object property has 3 sub properties that qualify the type of influence that is asserted. These are:

- Assert-Positive-Influencing-Factor: The property states that the `Evidence` confirms a significant positive `Influencingfactor`. Positive influence implies that the factor motivates good TAB. For example, `Study-001` ***assertPosInfFactor*** `HighIncome`
- Assert-Negative-Influencing-Factor: The property states that the `Evidence` confirms a significant negative `Influencingfactor`. Negative influence implies that the factor motivates poor TAB. For example, `Study-002` ***assertNegInfFactor*** `AlcoholAbuse`
- Assert-Neutral-Influencing-Factor: The property states that the `Evidence` confirms a neutral `Influencingfactor`. Neutral influence implies a non-significant or unknown influence of the factor. For example, `Study-010` ***assertNeuInfFactor*** `GoodExercise`

The above primitives provide further expressivity for modellers to qualify asserted factors, but this is not enforced, i.e. the `assertInfFactor` relation may still be used if the modeller wishes not to qualify the influence of a factor.

Study-evidence → Publication: `isPublishedAs`

The `isPublishedAs` relationship exists between a `Study` and a `Publication` that shows whether the study has been published as a research document. The relationship is represented with the `isPublishedAs` object property. For instance

> `SouthAfrica-001` ***isPublishedAs*** `CharacteristicsOfAnti-` `tuberculosisMedicationAdherenceInSouthAfrica.`

This relationship allows modellers to discover those influencing factors that are supported by published studies. The publication also serves as a reference for factors discovered by specific studies.

Study-evidence → Region: `hasRegion`

This relationship provides location information of the `Evidence`. This is very important for modellers to be able to link the assertions of factors to the region where the study is carried out. The relationship is represented by "`hasRegion`". Modellers can use the region of the study to look for factors that are within a particular region and base their models on factors asserted by studies in that region or in regions with profiles similar to their own.

3.3   Usage of the TAB Influencing Factor Ontology

Reasoning with the Evidence

The main purpose of the ontology is to specify a wide range of potential influencing factors, supported by published scientific studies. The modeller will then explore the ontology either by navigation or querying to discover and select potential factors that are appropriate for a specific community.

For instance, influencing factors can be selected based on the number of positive or negative influences that are asserted by previous studies. This provides an opportunity to fine tune the influencing factors' selected by modellers. For example, alcohol abuse may be a stronger negative influencing factor than unemployment as asserted by previous studies presented in the ontology. Lists of influencing factors can be generated and refined by location, number of supporting studies, year that the study was carried out, or cohort (sample) size.

Consider a scenario where a modeller wishes to find a set of potential influencing factors based on studies carried out on Ethiopian communities after 2009. First, the ontology is queried for influencing factors that have been asserted by any study. This is done by using the inverse of `assertInfFactor` object property. This query is shown in the Manchester OWL Syntax [25] below.

```
Class ExampleClass:

EquivalentTo: Factor and (infFactorAssertedBy some
               Evidence)
```

The query is then refined to reflect the study related assertions only and narrowed down by the region of the study.

```
Class ExampleClass:
EquivalentTo:  InfluencingFactor and (infFactorAs-
               sertedBy some (Study and hasRegion
               value Ethiopia))
```

Study size and year are two other constraints that can be used to restrict evidence. A modeller may intend to set a minimum sample size and only consider factors that are asserted by recent studies. A complete query for selecting factors that are identified by published studies carried out in Ethiopia from 2009 till date, which has a sample size not less than 500 patients is shown below:

```
Class ExampleClass:
EquivalentTo:  InfluencingFactor and (infFactorAssert-
               edBy some (Study and ((hasRegion value Ethio-
               pia) and (hasSampleSize some integer [>= 500])
               and (hasYear some integer [>=2009]) and (isPu-
               blishedAs some Publication))))
```

All the queries described above can be executed via the DL query tab in the Protégé tool.

Complex Class Creation from the Influencing Factor Ontology

Although the ontology is reasonably comprehensive, it can still be extended. The factor category can be extended either by creating a new main category or sub classes to the existing categories. Querying the factors and creating equivalent classes for the result of the queries can form new factor categories. This is important for creating classes that will be used for the construction of a DN in the event that the classes represented in the ontology do not match the community of interest.

For example, assuming we need to create a new class called "Personal Attitude" to represent groups of factors that are associated with TB patient's behaviour. This class will consist of some patient demographic information and some social related factors. The principle behind this derived class is that each patient has their normal daily attitude that contributes to their treatment adherence decision. The primary factors for this derived class are gender, age-group, emotion, depression, and stigma. The class is defined as:

```
Class Personal Attitude:
EquivalentTo:  Gender and MaritalStatus and
               AgeGroup and Emotion and Depression and
               Stigma
```

4 Construction of DN Model with the Ontology

The influencing factor ontology provides support for the construction of a DN model for TB adherence behaviour (TAB) for a specific community. A DN consists of two aspects, i.e. the network structure and the conditional probability table (CPT). The structure is composed of nodes and the arcs that represent the relationships between nodes. In this section we describe how the ontology can be used to develop the structure of an appropriate belief network (Bayesian network).

Firstly, a list of nodes and their respective states are generated from the ontology. Then, these nodes are linked with arcs to form a belief (Bayesian) network. The belief network is modified into a DN by adding decision and utility nodes. Lastly, CPT tables are added to each nodes based on the occurrence probability and influence weighting of each of the factors represented in the network.

4.1 Decision Model Development Methodology

An example case study is described below to explain the method for constructing the DN model. It demonstrates how modellers can use the ontology to construct a DN model for a specific TB community in sub-Saharan Africa.

Defining the Example Case

Suppose that a modeller wishes to develop a TAB DN for South Africa. By exploring the ontology, the modeller discovers a paper by Naidoo *et al.* [26]. The modeller discovered that five of the influencing factors identified by the paper are represented in the ontology. The factors, which are gender, age group, alcohol abuse, comorbidity and poverty level are useful and adequate to model a DN for his/her TB community. This is because the paper affirms that poor TAB are influenced by:

- Gender: Being a male patient
- Age-group: Patient with age above 34 years
- Alcohol abuse: Patients who abuse alcohol
- Comorbidity: Patient undertaking treatment for more than one chronic disease
- Poverty level: Patient with medium and high poverty level

The modeller decides to use these factors for modelling and testing an initial DN for his/her TB community. The modeller must select the relevant classes from the ontology and these will be automatically transformed into an appropriate belief network structure.

Selection of Relevant Classes (Factors)

The ontology was queried to select the list of influencing factors that are required to compose the list of the root nodes and their states. This was carried out by applying a query to identify the influencing factors identified by the study which was published as [26].

```
Class CaseStudy:
EquivalentTo: InfluencingFactor and (infFactorAssert-
     edBy some (Study and ((hasRegion value SouthAf-
     rica) and (isPublishedAs value PredictorsOf-
     TuberculosisAndAntiretroviralMedicationNon-
     adherenceInPublicPrimaryCarePatientsInSouthAf-
     rica-ACrossSectionalStudy))))
```

With the above query, the five influencing factor classes and their instances asserted by [26] are selected.

Transformation of Ontology Primitives into Belief Network Primitives

The TAB ontology is designed such that classes and instances in the ontology can be directly mapped to primitives in a belief network. The mapping is shown in Fig. 4 below.

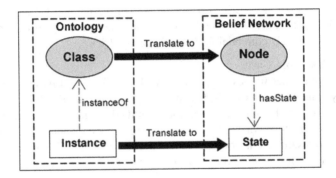

Fig. 4. Transformation of ontology primitives into belief network primitives

The selected factors from the ontology are transformed into nodes, and their respective instances translate into node states. In our example case, the five nodes generated are the root nodes of the belief network. For instance Age-group node and its three discrete states is a direct translation of the "AgeGroup" class and the instances "18-34", "35-44" and "Above 44". Table 1 below shows the influencing factor classes and their corresponding instances. The classes are needed to construct the root nodes to be linked to the hypothesis node (TAB).

Generating the Decision Network

While the (factor) nodes and states are dynamically generated from the ontology, the central TAB, and decision and utility nodes are static. All factor nodes become parent nodes of the TAB node, to form a Naïve Bayes network structure.

Figure 5 below shows the diagram of the DN model for the case study. The DN model consists of a TAB belief network. The influencing factors are modelled as root nodes. The TAB node is the hypothesis node; its states are the patient's TAB that determines the patient's decision to take the drugs. The "Take Drugs" node is a

Table 1. Selected influencing factors for the DN model

Class/Node	Instance/State
Gender	Male
	Female
AgeGroup	18–34
	35–44
	Above44
PovertyLevel	LowPoverty
	MediumPoverty
	HighPoverty
HIVComorbidity	Comorbidity-True
	Comorbidity-False
AlcoholAbuse	AlcoholAbuse-True
	AlcoholAbuse-False

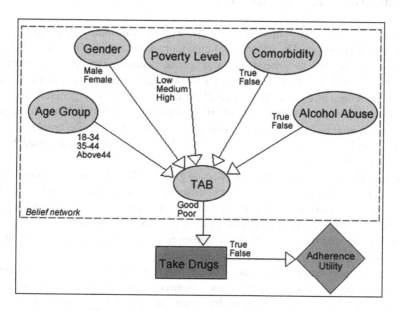

Fig. 5. Example case decision network model

decision node that is influenced by the TAB state of the patient. Adherence utility node measures the adherence risk of TB patients

With the structure in place, the modeller can do further customisation of the network, including refinement of the CPTs and adding additional nodes. While default CPTs are generated along with the structure, these must be repopulated by the modeller to adequately represent the target community, based on a combination of expert knowledge and data obtained from the target community. While the ontology provides some indication of the weighting of the influencing relation (negative, neutral or positive) determining CPT values is currently not addressed by the ontology and is left for future work.

Automation of the DN Construction with Tools
As described above an appropriate DN can be automatically generated from the ontology. An initial prototype was implemented in Java to automate the construction of the belief network model. Queries to extract classes and instances from the ontology were written in SPARQL and implemented using the Java Jena API[2].

The Jena API provided a platform for automating the transformation of the classes into node lists and the dependency information required to construct the network structure. The Bayesian network tool (BNJ) [27] was then used to generate an initial BN structure. Further customisation is carried out manually using the Hugin Expert[3] Bayesian network tool

5 Conclusions and Future Work

This paper presents an ontology to capture and consolidate knowledge about influencing factors for TB adherence behaviour. Furthermore, it shows how the ontology can be used to generate an appropriate decision network for a particular community. While Bayesian networks have been used previously to model adherence, to our knowledge, this is the first approach to use an ontology to generate the initial network structure. An important feature of the ontology is the integration of literature and scientific studies to support the inclusion of various factors. The ontology covers both the breadth and the depth of factors in sub-Saharan Africa as reported by key scientific review papers.

The ontology can be used by modellers to generate DNs for specific communities. Modellers may easily discover and select classes and their instances from the ontology which can be used to create the nodes and states of a belief network. A mechanism is proposed for direct translation from the ontology structure to the BN structure, to ease DN model construction. User specified influencing factor classes are translated into nodes while instances are converted into the states.

The expected impact of the study is to facilitate wider usage of decision support tools for TB patient management in low resource countries of sub-Saharan Africa. A decision network tool can be used by healthcare workers in identifying potential defaulters by generating risk indices for TB patients in a particular community. Allocation of resources, most especially scarce healthcare worker time, can be optimised based on risk levels in particular communities. This will help simplify TB patient monitoring and follow up services.

This study is a first step towards automating decision network construction with limited expert knowledge of TAB. Prior to this study, knowledge about TAB influencing factors were encapsulated in scientific publications and difficult to harmonise. The study

---

[2] https://jena.apache.org/.

[3] http://www.hugin.com/.

made successful attempt to harmonise the influencing factors from scientific publication and presented them as structured knowledge useful for predicting TAB amongst other possible uses.

The proposed ontology serves as a repository of TAB knowledge useful in high TB prevalence region like sub-Saharan Africa to support patient management. The repository of knowledge is very important to support public health decision making. It provides a possibility to share and reuse knowledge about influencing factors of TAB. The study is an important step towards providing a global repository of harmonised knowledge about TAB influencing factors.

However, there is the need for strengthening of the ontology for DN construction that is useful for prediction. This will involve the refinement of the ontology structure and the determination of the accuracy of input evidence in the ontology. There is also the need to improve the usefulness of the DN through the strengthening of the input information and the complexity of the network to represent patient's TAB in reality. The improved DN will be evaluated on usefulness to predict patient's TAB

Future work includes strengthening the `Evidence` class in the ontology, introduction of influence weighting for CPT generation, modelling spatial relation for `Region` class, and populating the ontology with more evidence from sub-Saharan African and other regions as well. Furthermore, TAB influencing factor ontology will also be presented as a web-service where users can query for influencing factors that represents their community of interest.

Development of complex DN models using the ontology is another direction to further explore. The TAB DN model will be developed to enhance its usefulness for patient management support. Lastly, our proposed method can be developed into a platform for predicting TB patient's behaviour in relation to treatment.

Acknowledgement. This work, including support for the Health Architecture Laboratory (HeAL) project as well as for DM, CS and AP and a PhD scholarship to KO, was funded by grants from the Rockefeller Foundation (Establishing a Health Enterprise Architecture Lab, a research laboratory focused on the application of enterprise architecture and health informatics to resource-limited settings, Grant Number: 2010 THS 347) and the International Development Research Centre (IDRC) (Health Enterprise Architecture Laboratory (HeAL), Grant Number: 106452-001). CS was additionally funded for aspects of this work by a grant from the Delegation of the European Union to South Africa to the South African Medical Research Council (SANTE 2007 147-790; Drug resistance surveillance and treatment monitoring network for the public sector HIV antiretroviral treatment programme in the Free State). The funders had no role in study design, data collection and analysis, decision to publish, or preparation of the manuscript.

References

1. WHO: Global tuberculosis report 2013, p. 145. World Health Organization, Geneva, Switzerland (2013)
2. Gandhi, N.R., Nunn, P., Dheda, K., Schaaf, H.S., Zignol, M., van Soolingen, D., Jensen, P., Bayona, J.: Multidrug-resistant and extensively drug-resistant tuberculosis: a threat to global control of tuberculosis. Lancet **375**(9728), 1830–1843 (2010)

3. Munro, S.A., Lewin, S.A., Smith, H.J., Engel, M.E., Fretheim, A., Volmink, J.: Patient adherence to tuberculosis treatment: a systematic review of qualitative research. Plos Med. **4**(7), 1230–1245 (2007)
4. Sabaté, E.: Organization WH: Adherence to Long-term Therapies: Evidence for Action: World Health Organization (2003)
5. CDC: Self-Study Modules on Tuberculosis: Patient Adherence to Tuberculosis Treatment. In. Edited by Prevention CfDCa, pp. 1–123. Centers for Disease Control and Prevention, Atlanta, Georgia (1999)
6. Mushlin, A.I., Appel, F.A.: Diagnosing potential noncompliance: physicians' ability in a behavioral dimension of medical care. Arch. Intern. Med. **137**(3), 318–321 (1977)
7. Costa, P.C., Laskey, K.B.: PR-OWL: a framework for probabilistic ontologies. Front. Artif. Intell. Appl. **150**, 237 (2006)
8. Laskey, K.B., Costa, P.C., Janssen, T.: Probabilistic ontologies for knowledge fusion. In: 11th International Conference on Information Fusion, pp. 1–8. IEEE (2008)
9. Rajput, Q.N., Haider, S.: Use of Bayesian network in information extraction from unstructured data sources. Int. J. Inf. Technol. **5**(4), 207–213 (2009)
10. Gruber, T.R.: Toward principles for the design of ontologies used for knowledge sharing. Int. J. Hum.-Comput. S.t **43**(5–6), 907–928 (1995)
11. Malhotra, A., Younesi, E., Gundel, M., Muller, B., Heneka, M.T., Hofmann-Apitius, M.: ADO: a disease ontology representing the domain knowledge specific to Alzheimer's disease. Alzheimer's & Dementia: J. Alzheimer's Assoc. **10**(2) (2013)
12. Alonso-Calvo, R., Maojo, V., Billhardt, H., Martin-Sanchez, F., Garcia-Remesal, M., Perez-Rey, D.: An agent- and ontology-based system for integrating public gene, protein, and disease databases. J. Biomed. Inform. **40**(1), 17–29 (2007)
13. Noy, N., McGuinness, D.: Ontology Development 101: A Guide to Creating Your First Ontology (2001)
14. Son, Y.J., Kim, H.G., Kim, E.H., Choi, S., Lee, S.K.: Application of support vector machine for prediction of medication adherence in heart failure patients. Healthcare Inform. Res. **16**(4), 253–259 (2010)
15. Dinh, T., Alperin, P.: A behavior-driven mathematical model of medication compliance. In: The 33rd Annual Meeting of the Society for Medical Decision Making. Society for Medical Decision Making (2011)
16. Nordmann, J.-P., Baudouin, C., Renard, J.-P., Denis, P., Regnault, A., Berdeaux, G.: Identification of noncompliant glaucoma patients using Bayesian networks and the eye-drop satisfaction questionnaire. Clin. Ophthalmol **4**, 1489–1496 (2010)
17. Cowell, L., Smith, B.: Infectious disease ontology. In: Sintchenko, V. (ed.) Infectious Disease Informatics, pp. 373–395. Springer, New York (2010)
18. Koum, G., Yekel, A., Ndifon, B., Etang, J., Simard, F.: Design of a two-level adaptive multi-agent system for malaria vectors driven by an ontology. BMC Med. Inform. Decis. Mak. **7**(1), 1–10 (2007)
19. Baker, P.G., Goble, C.A., Bechhofer, S., Paton, N.W., Stevens, R., Brass, A.: An ontology for bioinformatics applications. Bioinformatics **15**(6), 510–520 (1999)
20. Eilbeck, K., Jacobs, J., McGarvey, S., Vinion, C., Staes, C.: Exploring the use of ontologies and automated reasoning to manage selection of reportable condition lab tests from LOINC (2013)
21. Kostkova, P., Kumar, A., Roy, A., Madle, G., Carson, E.: Ontological Principles of Disease Management from Public Health Perspective: A Tuberculosis Case Study. City University, London (2005)

22. Dieng-Kuntz, R., Minier, D., Ruzicka, M., Corby, F., Corby, O., Alamarguy, L.: Building and using a medical ontology for knowledge management and cooperative work in a health care network. Comput. Biol. Med. **36**(7–8), 871–892 (2006)
23. Mabotuwana, T., Warren, J.: A framework for assessing adherence and persistence to long-term medication. Stud. Health Technol. Inform. **150**, 547–551 (2009)
24. Jin, J.J., Sklar, G.E., Min Sen Oh, V., Chuen Li, V.: Factors affecting therapeutic compliance: A review from the patient's perspective. Ther. Clin. Risk Manag. **4**(1), 269–286 (2008)
25. Horridge, M., Drummond, N., Goodwin, J., Rector, A.L., Stevens, R., Wang, H.: The Manchester OWL syntax. In: OWLed (2006)
26. Naidoo, P., Peltzer, K., Louw, J., Matseke, G., Mchunu, G., Tutshana, B.: Predictors of tuberculosis (TB) and antiretroviral (ARV) medication non-adherence in public primary care patients in South Africa: a cross sectional study. BMC Public Health **13**(1), 396 (2013)
27. Moodley, D., Simonis, I., Tapamo, J.R.: An architecture for managing knowledge and system dynamism in the worldwide sensor web. Int. J. Semant. Web Inf. Syst. **8**(1), 64–88 (2012)

From Requirements to Code:
Model Based Development
of a Medical Cyber Physical System

Anitha Murugesan[1]([✉]), Mats P.E. Heimdahl[1], Michael W. Whalen[1],
Sanjai Rayadurgam[1], John Komp[1], Lian Duan[1],
Baek-Gyu Kim[2], Oleg Sokolsky[2], and Insup Lee[2]

[1] Department of Computer Science and Engineering,
University of Minnesota, 200 Union Street, Minneapolis, MN 55455, USA
{anitha,heimdahl,whalen,rsanjai,komp,lduan}@cs.umn.edu
[2] Department of Computer and Information Science, University of Pennsylvania,
3330 Walnut Street, Philadelphia, PA 19104, USA
{baekgyu,sokolsky,lee}@cis.upenn.edu

Abstract. The advanced use of technology in medical devices has improved the way health care is delivered to patients. Unfortunately, the increased complexity of modern medical devices poses challenges for development, assurance, and regulatory approval. In an effort to improve the safety of advanced medical devices, organizations such as FDA have supported exploration of techniques to aid in the development and regulatory approval of such systems. In an ongoing research project, our aim is to provide effective development techniques and exemplars of system development artifacts that demonstrate state of the art development techniques.

In this paper we present an end-to-end model-based approach to medical device software development along with the artifacts created in the process. While outlining the approach, we also describe our experiences, challenges, and lessons learned in the process of formulating and analyzing the requirements, modeling the system, formally verifying the models, generating code, and executing the generated code in the hardware for generic patient controlled analgesic infusion pump (GPCA). We believe that the development artifacts and techniques presented in this paper could serve as a generic reference to be used by researchers, practitioners, and authorities while developing and evaluating cyber physical medical devices.

1 Introduction

Cyber Physical Systems (CPS) systems are physical systems whose operations are monitored and controlled by digital – often networked – computers. Advances in medical device technology, especially sophisticated software controls, has

This work has been partially supported by NSF grants CNS-0931931 and CNS-1035715.

M. Huhn and L. Williams (Eds.): FHIES 2014/SEHC 2014, LNCS 9062, pp. 96–112, 2017.
DOI: 10.1007/978-3-319-63194-3_7

improved health care delivery. Nevertheless, the increased use of software has lead to new failure modes for complex medical devices, for example, the numerous recalls on infusion pumps – a medical device used for controlled drug delivery to patients – indicate that they have posed serious health hazards [3]. Hence, along with the advances in technology comes the need for effective development and regulatory practices to ensure the safety of such systems. In an effort to improve the safety of advanced medical devices, organizations such as FDA have supported initiatives to aid in the development and regulatory approval of such systems, for example, the Infusion Pump Initiative [3]. Our aim is to contribute to these initiatives by defining and demonstrating effective development techniques, and providing archetypes of system development artifacts of a medical device.

In this paper, we describe an end-to-end model based approach for developing medical device software; we outline our approach, elaborate on our experiences, challenges, and lessons learned when formulating and analysing requirements, modeling the system, performing formal verification, generating code, and executing the generated code to control an infusion pump. We use a Generic Patient Controlled Analgesia Infusion Pump (GPCA) system – a type of infusion pump – to illustrate our approach. We believe that the development techniques and the artifacts presented can serve as a generic exemplar to be used by researchers, practitioners, and authorities while developing and evaluating these type of devices. All the artifacts discussed in this paper are available at http://crisys. cs.umn.edu/gpca.shtml.

The paper is organized as follows. Section 2 gives an overview of our model based development approach followed by Sect. 3 providing an overview of the GPCA system – the case example that is used throughout the paper. Section 4 describes the requirements analysis and modeling efforts. Section 5 provides an overview of the verification strategies including a discussion on how our specific GPCA implementation is analysed in context of a closed loop medical system. Section 6 discusses the hardware-code integration challenges. Finally Sect. 7 concludes with a brief summary of our work and the steps to the future.

2   A Model Based Development Approach

We advocate a model based approach to the development of CPS software. Model-based development allows the unambiguous capture of requirement, architecture, and design detail, and enables the extensive use of tools and automation. This allows for greatly reduced manual effort while maintaining or improving the capability of fault finding and enhancing quality of the system [14,15].

To ascertain that a system is safe and effective, it is imperative to precisely specify its requirements. In practice, however, the requirement are rarely (if ever) well known at the onset of a project. Instead, the initial set of requirements form a basis for a proposed solution (an initial systems architecture or design). In our case, we advocate modeling to evaluate design alternatives and explore the desired system. In effect, the models are proposed solutions to the problem at

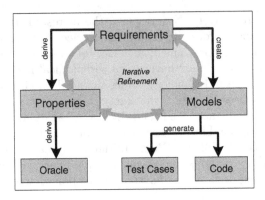

Fig. 1. Approach overview

hand (the requirements); the models are early prototypes of a proposed system that help visualize and analyse the problem as well as the proposed solution (Fig. 1).

Models and requirements exist in a symbiotic relationship; through iterative evolution they contribute to each other's improvement. While constructing models of a system – by exploring the solution domain – an engineer adds architectural and design detail not specifically stated in requirements, architectural and design information that helps clarify existing requirement as well as discover missing ones [6,27]. Similarly, as requirements are modified and added, the models evolve to accommodate the new constraints. Throughout the process, while modeling, one may find that the design cannot meet the system-level requirements (for example, the requirements may be unrealizable or there is no cost effective solution). This may lead to the imposition of constraints on the system's operational environment or a renegotiation of the system-level requirements. Nuseibeh identified this virtuous cycle as the Twin Peaks model [20]. If the modeling notation is formal, various verification techniques can be used to determine if formalized requirements (that is, desirable model properties) are satisfied in the model; a failed verification (the model does not meet the requirements) points to a problem that must be addressed through a modified model, modified requirements, or a further constrained operating environment. Miller et al. first advocated such a process in the context of developing critical avionics systems [14].

In addition to the advantages during the early development phases, a formal model-based approach can be leveraged throughout the life-cycle. Using commercial tools, the models and requirements can be used for code generation, test case generation, and used as oracles during testing. In the following sections we will discuss the various steps in the process and share the experiences we gained from developing artifacts for the Generic Patient Controlled Analgesia Infusion Pump (GPCA).

3   GPCA System Overview

Infusion pumps are medical CPS used for controlled delivery of liquid drugs into a patient's body according to a physician's *prescription*, a set of instructions that governs the plan of care for that individual. Modern infusion pumps have evolved to include several features for different drug delivery modes, programmability, notifications and logging. For instance, most pumps deliver the drug at a constant (and usually low) rate for an extended period of time, called *basal* delivery mode. Special types of pumps such as Patient-controlled analgesia (PCA) pumps are equipped with a feature that allows patients to self-administer a controlled amount of drug – a *patient bolus* mode may be activated to deliver prescribed additional drug, typically to alleviate acute pain. The pumps also have the capability to monitor and notify the clinicians when exceptional conditions such as air embolism occur, when they are in use.

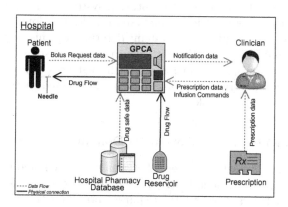

Fig. 2. GPCA overview

Figure 2 shows an external intravenous Generic Patient Controlled Analgesia (GPCA) device in a typical usage environment, a hospital or a clinic. A clinician, a certified practitioner, operates the GPCA device: programs the prescription information, loads the drug, connects the device with the patient, and responds to notifications from the device. The patient receives the drug from the device through an intravenous needle inserted by the clinician. The patient can self administer prescribed amounts of additional drug by pressing a bolus request button accessible at the patient's bed. The GPCA also has an interface to the hospital pharmacy repository for accessing manufacturer provided drug information that is typically used to verify if the programmed therapy regimen is within drug safe limits. The GPCA has three primary functions: (1) deliver the drug based on the prescribed schedule and patient requests, (2) prevent hazards that may arise during its usage, and (3) monitor and notify the clinician of certain exceptional conditions encountered. In our work we focus on analysing the infusion pump's software that controls the drug infusion and raises alarms to notify the clinician when hazards are detected. Other infusion pump subsystems such as the user interface, sensors and actuators are out of scope of this work.

4   Model Based Requirements Analysis

As mentioned in Sect. 2, it is imperative to have a well defined set of requirement for a system that is discovered through deliberations between stakeholders. Effective requirements elicitation relies on an iterative process where the requirement domain and the solution space are explored concurrently [20]. In our work, early system modeling and analysis have served as crucial aids. Nevertheless, during the requirements and modeling efforts of the GPCA, several challenges – some unexpected, some expected – with developing requirements for CPS surfaced. First, in CPS, the system level requirements are expressed in the physical world; discovering, understanding, and capturing these requirements were unexpectedly challenging. Second, closely related to capturing system level requirements is the determination of what is considered the system under development and what is considered the environment of the system; determining this system boundary was an unexpected challenge. Finally, even a simple system contains several interacting features; properly understanding the patterns of interaction among features (the feature interaction problem) was an expected challenge where our modeling efforts were invaluable.

4.1   Requirements in the Continuous Domain

Understanding the interaction patterns between the system and its environment as well as between the various hardware and software components within the system is crucial for capturing CPS requirements. The behavior of both the hardware components as well as the environment is continuous and continual in nature. Frequently, we found that the requirements for a system were focusing on the ordering of events in the system (as is done with various temporal logics) and the real-time constraints on these events. That information, however, is not sufficient to capture the continuous and continual nature of the system. For example, the rate of change of a controlled variable, the time it takes for a controlled variable to settle sufficiently close to a set-point, and the cumulative errors built up over time may be of critical importance, concepts that we found were not stated explicitly as requirements. For example, let us consider a safety requirement of the GPCA,

> *"An over-infusion alarm shall be triggered if the flow rate of the drug in the infusion tubing is greater than X% of the prescribed flow rate for more than Y minutes"*

This requirement concerns the response to a flow rate of drug exceeding the prescribed value. Nevertheless, a closer examination of the problem reveals some ambiguity: Is it acceptable for the flow rate to exceed the threshold for Y

consecutive minutes or does the time accumulate over the full infusion interval? Similarly, what is the cumulative effect of excess drug flow? For example, if the flow periodically exceeds $X\%$ for $Y-1$ consecutive minutes and then comes back to normal for a short period of time, there is a possibility of over-infusion due the rate at which the drug is infused as well as the overall volume infused into the patient within a certain interval of time. We found behavioral modeling in the physical domain particularly useful in the elicitation, discovery, and refinement of such requirements.

Control System Modeling: To understand the control behavior of the system in the continuous domain, we developed control system models – traditionally used to evaluate various control strategies, tune the controllers, etc.

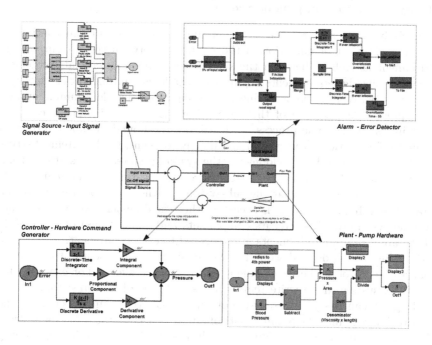

Fig. 3. Control system model

For the GPCA, we developed these models using MathWorks Simulink [12] tools to better understand the requirements needed to adequately constrain the desired system behavior (Fig. 3) [6]. Through these modeling efforts we had an opportunity to explore various system responses, investigate how a proposed system might behave in its intended environment, and thereby identify precise requirements for the system. For example, the overinfusion safety requirement is now refined and stated as,

"The software shall issue an over-infusion alarm if the flow rate of the drug in the infusion tubing is greater than X% of the prescribed flow rate

for more than Y consecutive minutes or more than Z minutes cumulative during the infusion duration."
"The software shall issue an over-infusion alarm if the volume of drug delivered in P consecutive minutes anytime during the infusion duration is more than Q% of the prescribed volume to be infused in that interval."

Through this modeling exercise, in addition to identifying precise requirements for the software, we were also able to identify categories of requirements that should be considered while capturing requirements for a cyber physical system, for example, accuracy, rise/drop time, rate of change, overshoot or maximum deviation, settling time, and cumulative error [6].

4.2   System and Component Scope

To precisely state requirements such as the requirements of the continuous domain, a clear-cut demarcation of the boundary between the system and its environment as well as between the system components is crucial. Scoping a system is a classic requirements engineering challenge and insufficient analysis among and between different engineering disciplines when determining system scope (precise demarcation of the system boundary) is a significant cause of CPS failures [10,24]. The process of identifying the boundary is not restricted to the interface between the system and its environment; the hierarchical structure of the system under development (the system architecture) is also crucial. Most systems are developed as collections of communicating smaller, manageable sub-systems. To ascertain that the sub-systems – when composed – satisfy the overall system requirements, it is necessary that the designers express the structure (the system architecture, its components and connections) of the system and the appropriate requirements are allocated to each component.

Providing a well defined scope for the requirements is essential to maintain intellectual control of the development and assurance efforts. For example, for the GPCA system, if we write requirements in terms of the *prescribed dosage* of a drug, we can postpone discussion of entry errors (the clinician entering the prescribed dosage into the pump is part of our system). On the other hand, from a development perspective, it is most likely preferable to write infusion pump requirements in terms of the *dosage entered at the pump interface*; the clinician is not part of the pump system and entry errors are part of its environment. Thus, the choice of scope does not only have implications for our development efforts (what is "in" our system and what is "outside" our system), but also has profound implications for the way the system is assured for safety.

To assist us in the process of scoping the GPCA system and establishing rigorous interfaces between the system and its environment as well as between system components we relied on architectural modeling. The scoping exercise forced us to consistently express requirements in terms of inputs and outputs at a particular level of abstraction.

Architectural Models: For the GPCA, we developed an architectural model, shown in Fig. 4[1], that clearly defines its interfaces (input and output variables) [17]. We used the Architecture Analysis and Description Language (AADL) [23] for the modeling. For formal verification (discussed in Sect. 5), the GPCA turned out to be too large to be handled as a monolithic model; hence to manage complexity and maintain intellectual control, we decomposed it into smaller manageable components and defined an architecture that specified how the components are connected. The architecture also clearly specifies the interfaces of each component. This exercise typically occurs repeatedly over several layers of system abstraction; each component in the architectural model has its own set of interfaces, subcomponents, and component requirements. Rigorously defining the interfaces helped consistently scope all requirements by expressing them strictly in terms of the respective interface variables. The choice of the system boundary (the scope of the system) for a requirements effort is of course debatable; in our work we do not attempt to suggest an optimal scope. We would like, however, to emphasize that whatever scope boundary is chosen, it must be well defined and all requirements and environmental assumptions must be stated based on this system boundary [4].

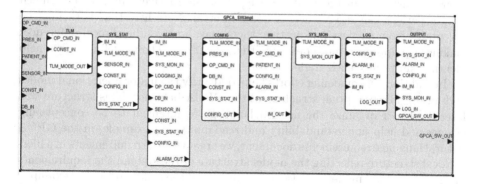

Fig. 4. Architectural model

4.3 Mode Logic Requirements

Although the architectural models helped to clarify the interfaces to ease the requirements definition burden, they do not help resolve the complexity of the behavioral requirements on the system. The dynamic behaviors of complex systems are frequently defined in terms of operational *modes*, which are frequently viewed to be mutually exclusive sets of system behaviors [11]. The modes together with the rules defining the transitions between them are called *mode logic* [8]. Derivation of precise requirements of the mode logic is challenging due to the plurality of modes and the complexity of the rules that govern the

---

[1] In Fig. 4, the connections between components are abstracted for visual clarity.

transitions. In the GPCA, understanding the mode logic of the various infusion delivery types, such as basal or bolus, was nontrivial and we again relied on modeling to illuminate and resolve the issues.

Finite State Machine Models: To analyze the GPCA infusion mode logic requirements and behaviors, we modeled it as a finite state machine, using Math-Works' Simulink and Stateflow [12]. A portion of the model of the GPCA infusion mode logic is shown in Fig. 5. In our endeavor to model the mode logic [16], we identified requirements and modeling patterns and requirement scenarios not apparent before the modelling efforts.

For example, a statement from one of the versions of the GPCA software's requirements document reads:

> *"A patient bolus shall take precedence over a square bolus. At the completion of the patient bolus, the square bolus shall continue delivery."*

This requirement may be taken to mean that the patient bolus simply overrides the programmed square bolus infusion as illustrated in Fig. 6(a) or the square bolus is suspended until the patient bolus is delivered and resumed thereafter as illustrated in Fig. 6(b). Clearly, these alternatives influence how much drug a patient can receive over a bolus interval. Note here that both may be acceptable from a safety perspective; there may, however, be clinical differences making one approach more desirable than the other. The modeling efforts help identify and resolve such tradeoffs.

In addition, the modeling efforts helped identify the major operational modes and an overall conceptual structure of the GPCA behavior. This structure was later used to reorganize the natural language requirement to be conceptually cleaner and help understandability and readability. For example, in the GPCA natural language requirements document, we organized the requirements in a hierarchical structure reflecting the model structure of the system; the requirements of the parent level modes are also applicable to all the child modes. For example,

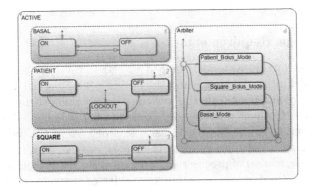

Fig. 5. Infusion mode logic of GPCA

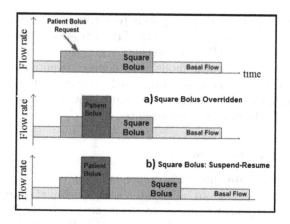

Fig. 6. Mode interaction patterns

all requirements applicable for the Active mode are also applicable in the Basal mode (submode of Active). This organization enhanced clarity and reduced the repetition of a requirement in multiple places within the same document.

5   Formal Verification

As mentioned previously, complex systems are hierarchically constructed. For example, the GPCA software was decomposed into several components (captured in the AADL architectural model), requirements allocated to each component, and the detailed functionality of each component captured in the behavioral model (captured using Simulink and Stateflow). Thus, to verify the system as a whole, one needs a verification chain to help determine (1) whether or not the composition – based on the architecture – of the component level requirements is adequate to establish the system-level requirements, (2) if the detailed specification of a component's behavior satisfy the component-level requirements, and (3) whether the system operating in its intended environment will meet the safety constraints defined in the physical world. In this section, we summarize our verification strategy. A more detailed account is available in previous publications [19].

5.1   Compositional Verification

To formally prove that a system decomposed into an architecture satisfies its system level requirements requires a compositional argument involving (i) the component behaviors and (ii) the assumptions about the system's environment [5]. To perform compositional verification of the GPCA, we used AGREE (Assume Guarantee Reasoning Environment) – a compositional verification framework developed for AADL verification [2]. AGREE is based on assume-guarantee reasoning [13], that provides an appropriate mechanism for formally capturing the component requirements, and assumptions to verify system requirements. The AGREE framework is a plugin to the OSATE environment (the same environment used to model the AADL architecture).

In the GPCA architectural model, we defined requirements as assume-guarantee contracts for each component, as well as for the system as a whole. The AGREE tool automatically verifies if the component contracts in the specified architecture satisfy the system requirements.

5.2   Behavioral Verification

Knowing that the architecture and component requirements meet the system level requirement, it remains to be shown that the detailed component specifications meet the component requirement. As mentioned in the previous section, the component behaviours were modeled using MathWorks Simulink and Stateflow tools. Hence, using MathWorks Simulink Design Verifier (SDV) [12] – a plug-in tool for formal verification – one can verify that the behavioral models satisfy requirements modeled as synchronous observers. Ideally, the component requirements captured in AGREE would be reused as synchronous observers in the verification of the component behaviors. Unfortunately, the automatic translation from AGREE contracts to a notation acceptable in the Simulink Design Verifier has not been completed. Therefore, we manually translated the AGREE contracts to Embedded MATLAB. Embedded MATLAB was chosen over other possible notations (such as Simulink or Stateflow) for the observers since it is quite similar to the AGREE contracts making the translation easy. In the process of capturing the observers, we developed a structuring pattern for the Simulink and Stateflow models that would allow the independent evolution of the detailed behavioral models and the requirements captured as observers [26]. Given that the models of the GPCA had been decomposed into manageable pieces (through a combination of the compositional verification in AGREE and the component verification in SDV) scalability of the verification was not a problem and the overall correctness with respect to the system level requirements could be automatically established.

5.3   Verification in Context

Although one through compositional verification can demonstrate that the GPCA meets its requirements, this is no guarantee that the GPCA will work as intended in its operational environment. Thus, determining how the GPCA will perform when infusing a drug into a patient is of critical importance (Fig. 7).

In prior work, we verified a collection of safety properties of a closed-loop medical system in which an infusion pump is used to deliver opioid medication. A serious side effect of opioid medication is that overinfusion of the drug can lead to respiratory failure in patients. Hence a sensor, such as a pulse oximeter, used to detect onset of respiratory problems with patients, and a safety interlock device, that monitors the sensor readings, is used to command the pump to stop once a certain sensor reading (threshold) is crossed.

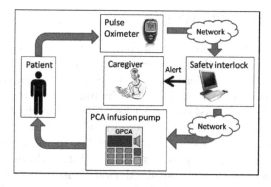

Fig. 7. GPCA in closed loop system

The closed loop system considered a highly abstract PCA pump [21] and was modeled as a timed automaton in UPPAAL [1] whereas the GPCA discussed in this paper is a detailed model of a realistic infusion pump with rich functionality captured in AGREE and Simulink/Stateflow. To demonstrate that the GPCA satisfies the closed loop real-time safety requirements, it is necessary to demonstrate that the GPCA (expressed in AGREE) satisfies the PCA requirement (captured in UPPAAL). For example, a closed loop system level requirement for the PCA informally states, *Infusion cannot begin until parameters of the infusion are configured and pump is started by the caregiver.* This requirement (continuous time), that was modeled as an automaton in UPPAAL, was recaptured as AGREE contracts as shown below. The first contract specifies that, at startup the system shall not be in the infusing mode and the second contract specifies that if `Infusion_Start` and `Infusion_Programmed` commands are not issued by the caregiver, the system shall not be in infusing mode. In the second contract `pre(PUMP_DISPLAY_OUT.Current_System_Mode)` indicates the value of the system mode in the previous execution step. These contracts were compositionally verified using the detailed GPCA's models by devising an informal abstraction mapping between the models [18].

```
property start_up_behaviour =
    is_start_up => (PUMP_DISPLAY_OUT.Current_System_Mode !="Infusing");

property no_infusion_start =
  true -> pre(PUMP_DISPLAY_OUT.Current_System_Mode) != "Infusing" and
    not(CAREGIVER_IN.Infusion_Start and CAREGIVER_IN.Infusion_Programmed)
    => (PUMP_DISPLAY_OUT.Current_System_Mode != "Infusing");
```

When attempting to perform compositional reasoning in a situation involving multiple modeling formalisms, verification paradigms, and associated tools, care must be taken to ensure that results from one formalism can be used in another formalism. To perform this verification, we employed a semi-formal approach for determining whether the results in UPPAAL could be composed with the results obtained in AGREE.

6   GPCA Implementation

The goal of a development project is of course to produce executable code that safely can be deployed on the target platform, in our case, a working infusion pump. Given our verified models, we relied on Simulink Coder [12] to automatically generate C code from the models. (The Simulink Coder is not a trusted code generator; thus, the generated code must be subjected to rigorous conformance testing demonstrating that no faults were introduced in the code generation. This testing is outside the scope of this paper but in can be fully automated as extensively discussed in our previous work [7,22,25]) Although the process of code generation from the model is straightforward, installing the software on the actual hardware can be a challenge. Below we discuss the challenges we faced while integrating the device with the generated code and discuss the approaches we took to address them.

6.1   Device Set up

Our target platform was a modified commercial infusion pump developed in the GPCA reference implementation project [9]. The experimental platform is a Baxter PCA infusion pump and is equipped with sensors and actuators that are necessary to verify infusion scenarios. The pump-motor (Fig. 8-(1)) is used to generate forces to move the loaded syringe downward, so that drug flows into a patient's body through the intravenous needle. The low and empty reservoir switches (Fig. 8-(2) and (3)) are used to detect if the remaining volume of drug in the syringe is too low or empty respectively. The patient bolus request button (Fig. 8-(4)) enables the patient to request an additional bolus dose. The door sensor (Fig. 8-(5)) is used to detect whether the door of the pump is opened or closed in order to prevent accidental removal of syringes during infusion. The buzzer (Fig. 8-(6)) is used to raise an audible signal when certain alarming condition occurs. These sensors and actuators are interfaced with a micro-controller board where the generated code from the model runs.

6.2   Hardware Abstractions and Code Clarity

The formal models describe the functionality of the system but abstract away hardware details such the signals needed to communicate with devices such as motors or buttons. Such abstraction is desirable to make the models device and hardware independent allowing us to target multiple physical infusion pumps with our generated code. On the other hand, it necessitates manually developed device dependent drivers to be provided with the generated code; thus, introducing a source of potential faults. Nevertheless, although in this project they were not developed, verified and trusted device drivers could be developed using the same techniques discussed throughout this paper.

Surprisingly, one of the most challenging aspects of the implementation effort was the task of understanding the generated code and identifying the appropriate signals within the model and connect them to the device drivers. This problem

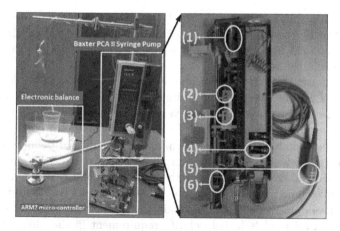

Fig. 8. Test setup with the Baxter Hardware (1) Pump Motor (2) Low Reservoir Switch (3) Empty Reservoir Switch (4) Door Sensor (5) Patient Bolus Request Button (6) Buzzer

can be largely attributed to our unfamiliarity with the code generator; simple tools support to assist in this endeavour would have been helpful and will be developed for our future case studies.

6.3   Testing the Code

Testing of the software on the target platform (as opposed to in the host environment on a workstation) brought new – although not entirely unexpected – challenges and insights. For example, we found that the variable recording the volume of remaining drug in the drug reservoir occasionally (and inexplicably) indicated that the reservoir had been refilled although no such action had been taken. In the model, this variable was defined as an unsigned 8-bit integer value; in the code, this variable was decremented below zero and a wrap-around occurred. One may wonder why this problem was not identified in any of the formal verification performed on the GPCA models. Although the problem led to unexpected behaviors, none of the behaviors violated the safety requirement that were the focus of the verification efforts. Note here that the Simulink Design Verifier has the capability of checking for under and overflow, in our initial verification efforts this capability was simply not used. Flaws such as this point to an inherent limitation of formal verification – the verification will only guarantee compliance with the properties actually used in the verification. Methods and techniques to help ensure that the set of requirements used in the verification is sufficient is an area needing further investigation.

7   Summary and Conclusion

In this paper we presented a model based development technique for developing critical cyber physical medical device systems. We illustrated our approach using a Generic Patient Controller Analgesia (GPCA) pump as a case study. While illustrating the approach ranging from natural language requirements to executable software, we also discussed some of the challenges we faced at the various stages in the project.

The intent with the GPCA development was as an exercise to develop and demonstrate effective development techniques and make the artifacts created in the process (requirements, models, verification properties, executable code, etc.) available publicly as exemplars. In the course of the project, there were several unexpected challenges, for example, the difficulty of defining the scope of a system (what is part of the system and what is part of the environment) and properly defining requirement for the continuous and real-time aspect of a system. To overcome these problems, we adopted a model based approach relying on the development of numerous models to address the challenges at hand: continuous control models to help clarify requirement in the physical domain, timed automata to verify closed loop properties of the infusion system, architectural models in AADL to help clarify system boundaries and explore the solution space, formal models of component contracts to verify that the architecture met system requirement, and detailed behavioral models of the components for verification and code generation. The generated code was integrated on multiple infusion pump hardware platforms to validate that the approach was feasible.

Following these efforts, we in this project will continue to develop the formal verification capabilities, explore the challenging questions related to rigorously and in an automated fashion test software in an embedded target environment, and explore how to perform verification in the inherently stochastic environment present in any cyber physical system.

References

1. Behrmann, G., David, A., Larsen, K.G.: A tutorial on UPPAAL. In: Bernardo, M., Corradini, F. (eds.) SFM-RT 2004. LNCS, vol. 3185, pp. 200–236. Springer, Heidelberg (2004). doi:10.1007/978-3-540-30080-9_7
2. Cofer, D., Gacek, A., Miller, S., Whalen, M.W., LaValley, B., Sha, L.: Compositional verification of architectural models. In: Goodloe, A.E., Person, S. (eds.) NFM 2012. LNCS, vol. 7226, pp. 126–140. Springer, Heidelberg (2012). doi:10.1007/978-3-642-28891-3_13
3. FDA. White Paper: Infusion Pump Improvement Initiative, April 2010
4. Gunter, C.A., Gunter, E.L., Jackson, M., Zave, P.: A reference model for requirements and specifications. IEEE Software 17(3), 37–43 (2000)
5. Hammond, J., Rawlings, R., Hall, A.: Will it work? [requirements engineering]. In: Fifth IEEE International Symposium on Requirements Engineering, Proceedings, pp. 102–109 (2001)
6. Heimdahl, M.P.E., Duan, L., Murugesan, A., Rayadurgam, S.: Modeling and requirements on the physical side of cyber-physical systems. In: Second International Workshop on the Twin Peaks of Requirements and Architecture, May 2013
7. Heimdahl, M.P.E., Rayadurgam, S., Visser, W., Devaraj, G., Gao, J.: Auto-generating test sequences using model checkers: a case study. In: 3rd International Workshop on Formal Approaches to Testing of Software (FATES 2003) (2003)

8. Joshi, A., Miller, S.P., Heimdahl, M.P.E.: Mode confusion analysis of a flight guidance system using formal methods. In: Proceedings of 22nd Digital Avionics Systems Conference (DASC 2003), vol. 1, p. 2-D. IEEE (2003)

9. Kim, B.G., Ayoub, A., Sokolsky, O., Lee, I., Jones, P., Zhang, Y., Jetley, R.: Safety-assured development of the GPCA infusion pump software. In: Proceedings of the International Conference on Embedded Software (EMSOFT), pp. 155–164, October 2011

10. Knight, J.C.: Safety critical systems: challenges and directions. In: Proceedings of the 24th International Conference on Software Engineering, pp. 547–550. IEEE (2002)

11. Leveson, N., Pinnel, L.D., Sandys, S.D., Koga, S., Reese, J.D.: Analyzing software specifications for mode confusion potential. In: Proceedings of a Workshop on Human Error and System Development, pp. 132–146 (1997)

12. MathWorks Inc. Products. http://www.mathworks.com/products

13. McMillan, K.L.: Circular compositional reasoning about liveness. Technical report 1999–02, Cadence Berkeley Labs, Berkeley, CA 94704 (1999)

14. Miller, S.P., Tribble, A.C., Whalen, M.W., Heimdahl, M.P.E.: Proving the shalls: early validation of requirements through formal methods. Int. J. Softw. Tools Technol. Transf. **8**(4), 303–319 (2006)

15. Miller, S.P., Whalen, M.W., Cofer, D.D.: Software model checking takes off. Commun. ACM **53**(2), 58–64 (2010)

16. Murugesan, A., Rayadurgam, S., Heimdahl, M.P.E.: Modes, features, and state-based modeling for clarity and flexibility. In: Fifth International Workshop on Modeling in Software Engineering, May 2013

17. Murugesan, A., Rayadurgam, S., Heimdahl, M.P.E.: Using models to address challenges in specifying requirements for medical cyber-physical systems. In: Fourth workshop on Medical Cyber-Physical Systems, April 2013

18. Murugesan, A., Sokolsky, O., Rayadurgam, S., Whalen, M., Heimdahl, M.P.E., Lee, I.: Linking abstract analysis to concrete design: a hierarchical approach to verify medical CPS safety. In: International Conference on Cyber-Physical Systems (ICCPS) 2014, April 2014

19. Murugesan, A., Whalen, M.W., Rayadurgam, S., Heimdahl, M.P.E.: Compositional verification of a medical device system. In: ACM International Conference on High Integrity Language Technology (HILT). ACM, November 2013

20. Nuseibeh, B.: Weaving together requirements and architectures. Computer **34**, 115–117 (2001)

21. Pajic, M., Mangharam, R., Sokolsky, O., Arney, D., Goldman, J., Lee, I.: Model-driven safety analysis of closed-loop medical systems. IEEE Trans. Ind. Inform. **PP**, 1–12 (2010). In early online access

22. Rajan, A., Whalen, M.W., Staats, M., Deng, W., Heimdahl, M.P.E.: The effect of program and model structure on the fault finding ability of MC/DC test suites. In: Proceedings of Int'l Symposium on Software Testing and Analysis (ISSTA) (2008, submitted). http://crisys.cs.umn.edu/ISSTA08.pdf

23. SAE. http://www.aadl.info/aadl/downloads/papers/aadllanguagesummary.pdf

24. Sha, L., Gopalakrishnan, S., Liu, X., Wang, Q.: Cyber-physical systems: a new frontier. In: Machine Learning in Cyber Trust, pp. 3–13. Springer, New York (2009)

25. Staats, M., Gay, G., Whalen, M.W., Heimdahl, M.P.E.: On the danger of coverage directed test case generation. In: 15th International Conference on Fundamental Approaches to Software Engineering (FASE), April 2012

26. Whalen, M., Murugesan, A., Rayadurgam, S., Heimdahl, M.: Structuring Simulink models for verification and reuse. In: Proceedings of the 6th International Workshop on Modeling in Software Engineering (2014)
27. Whalen, M.W., Gacek, A., Cofer, D., Murugesan, A., Heimdahl, M.P.E., Rayadurgam, S.: Your what is my how: iteration and hierarchy in system design. IEEE Software **30**(2), 54–60 (2013)

Demonstrating that Medical Devices Satisfy User Related Safety Requirements

Michael D. Harrison[1,4]([⊠]), Paolo Masci[2,3], Jose Creissac Campos[2,3], and Paul Curzon[1]

[1] School of Electronic Engineering and Computer Science,
Queen Mary University of London, Mile End, London E1 4NS, UK
michael.harrison@ncl.ac.uk
[2] Dep. Informática, Universidade do Minho, Braga, Portugal
[3] HASLab, INESC TEC, Braga, Portugal
[4] School of Computing Science, Newcastle University,
Newcastle upon Tyne NE1 7RU, UK

Abstract. One way of contributing to a demonstration that a medical device is acceptably safe is to show that the device satisfies a set of requirements known to mitigate hazards. This paper describes experience using formal techniques to model an IV infusion device and to prove that the modelled device captures a set of requirements. The requirements chosen for the study are based on a draft proposal developed by the US Food and Drug Administration (FDA). A major contributor to device related errors are (user) interaction errors. For this reason the chosen models and requirements focus on user interface related issues.

Keywords: Human error · Formal verification · Performance · Medical devices · Model checking · MAL · Theorem proving · PVS

1 Introduction

Regulators in diverse domains, including Aviation, Power Generation and Medicine, are tasked to ensure that system or device developers demonstrate that risks associated with the device are minimal or "as low as reasonably practicable". This must be done before the system or device can be deployed in a safety critical context. Such a demonstration can involve proving that the device satisfies a set of safety requirements designed to mitigate identified hazards (see [12]). The FDA has produced one such set of requirements in draft documentation [2] with a focus on medical devices, particularly infusion pumps. This paper is concerned with how to demonstrate that a device satisfies requirements, emphasising those that are *user related*. FDA guidelines propose that validation is "highly dependent upon comprehensive software testing, inspections, analyses and other verification tasks performed at each stage of the software development cycle" [19]. The data produced for such validation is usually substantial. The problem with testing (as has been noted often) is that it does not prove the absence of bugs.

© Springer International Publishing AG 2017
M. Huhn and L. Williams (Eds.): FHIES 2014/SEHC 2014, LNCS 9062, pp. 113–128, 2017.
DOI: 10.1007/978-3-319-63194-3_8

Formal techniques provide additional information. They are concise, precise and exhaustive. However they have the disadvantage that, with currently available tools, they are not easy to use although this situation is improving.

This paper demonstrates the use of formal techniques to provide assurance that a user related subset of the FDA requirements are met by an IV infusion pump. A formal model of the pump is used to prove properties that capture these requirements. The paper describes the steps taken to demonstrate that the requirements are satisfied. These steps include demonstrating that: the model is a faithful representation of the device; the chosen requirements are equivalent to the proved properties; and that the properties are true of the model. The paper aims to illustrate the approach without dwelling on detail to indicate its feasibility and progresses an agenda suggested by the FDA's use of formal techniques [11]. Section 2 sketches the infusion pump example. Sections 3, 4 and 5 are concerned with issues associated with producing a model that is a faithful representation of the device to be assessed. Section 6 suggests formalisations of the requirements that were used as a basis for proof. Section 7 briefly explores the proofs that were produced. The final section offers discussion and conclusions.

2   The Medical Example

The chosen device (the Alaris GP infusion pump [4] — see Fig. 1) has characteristics that are common to many devices that control processes over time. The clinician user sets infusion pump parameters and monitors the infusion process using the device. A model of the particular pump had already been developed [8][1] as part of a general analysis of usability properties of the device. The Alaris GP has two basic modes (besides the off mode): infusing and holding. These each have sub-modes. In the infusing mode the volume to be infused (vtbi) is pumped into the patient intravenously according to an infusion rate. In infusing mode the vtbi can be exhausted, in which case the pump continues in KVO (Keep Vein Open) mode and sets off an alarm. In holding mode the device is not infusing and values and settings can be changed. The complexity of the interface to this device is mainly concerned with values and settings that can be changed using a combination of function keys and chevron buttons (see Fig. 1). A subset of these features can also be changed when infusing. Chevron keys are used to increase (fup/sup), or decrease (fdown/sdown), entered numbers incrementally. Holding the chevron key down may have the effect of accelerating the size of the increment or decrement. The current data entry mode governs whether the chevron buttons can be used to change infusion rate, vtbi and time, or alternatively allow the user to move between options in a menu, for example in bag mode and in query mode. Bag mode allows the user to select from a set of infusion bag options, thereby setting vtbi to a predetermined value. Query mode, invoked by the query button, generates a menu of options. These can be configured by the manufacturer. Options include locking the infusion rate, disabling the locking of it, setting vtbi and time rather than vtbi and infusion rate, and changing the

---

[1] The models can be found at http://hcispecs.di.uminho.pt.

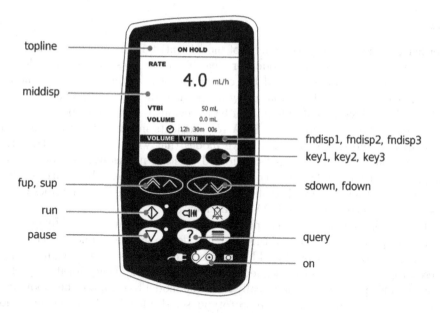

Fig. 1. Actions and attributes used to model the Alaris pump

units of volume and infusion rate. The device allows movement between display modes via three function keys (*key1*, *key2* and *key3*). Each function key has a display associated with it indicating its present function (*fndisp1*, *fndisp2* and *fndisp3*).

3   Modelling Infusion Devices: Background and Approach

3.1   Background

Safety requirements can be proved of a device through formal development by refining the model using tools such as Event B [1]. An initial model is first developed that specifies the device characteristics and incorporates the safety requirements. This initial model is gradually and iteratively refined, preserving the safety requirements, using details about how specific functionalities are implemented. Alternatively a model could be generated from the code of an existing device, using a set of transformation rules that guarantee correctness, as discussed in [10]. This approach has been demonstrated for the number entry components of an infusion pump, see [15].

Proving requirements has been the focus of previous work. For example, a mature set of tools have been developed by Heitmeyer's team using SCR [9]. Their approach uses a tabular notation to describe requirements which makes the technique relatively acceptable to developers. Combining simulation with model checking has also been a focus in, for example, [7]. Recent work concerned with simulations of PVS specifications provides valuable support to this complementarity [14].

3.2   The Approach

Neither refinement and development of models satisfying requirements nor producing models from program code were feasible in the present case. The device had already been developed and the code was not available to us. The model was therefore developed *by hand* using a combination of user manuals, simulations and the device itself. The model had previously been developed for other purposes, without the particular FDA requirements in mind. It had been used to analyse properties of the interactive modes that were described in the previous section. This analysis had considered whether modes were supported by the device without ambiguity, see [8]. For the presently described purpose this model was further developed to allow analysis of the details of the number entry system required to prove the FDA requirements.

Fidelity of the model to the implemented device was demonstrated by proving a range of properties. States of the modelled device were examined by comparing the traces of actions produced by the model checker, as counter-examples for these properties, with actual sequences generated by the device itself. A prototype was also produced automatically from the model to compare the "look and feel" of the actual device with the prototype, see [14] for details. The traces and simulations were indistinguishable from the behaviour of the physical device. The only difference between the simulation and the device was that no drug was infused, no connection was made to the patient and the precise timings differed. The simulations were generated with the aim that they could be explored by regulator or manufacturer. It is of course the case that they only allow an exploration of the paths that the regulator chooses to explore. Simulation can also be used to illustrate what the failure of a property means. Part of the argument to the regulator that this is acceptable may then involve a demonstration of the features of the device that fail the requirement, showing that they do not present a risk.

3.3   Modelling and Analysis of the Infusion Pump

The process of proving FDA requirements described in this paper involves a sequence of steps. These are as follows.

1. *Developing a model of the device.* Modelling involves two stages. First a version is produced to be analysed using model checking. Second the model is transformed systematically into a form to be analysed using theorem proving.
2. *Validating the model against the physical device.* This is done using a combination of plausibility properties and simulation based on the model.
3. *Formalising the requirements.* This involves two stages. The first stage disambiguates the requirement in a form that can be transformed into a device specific property. This formalisation is described in more detail in [13]. The second stage involves refining the formalised requirement to be specifically about the Alaris device. This process is typically interactive and in principle involves discussion with both human factors specialists, checking the validity

of the interpretation of the user-related requirement, and regulator to check that the property captures the spirit of the original requirement.

4. *Proving the property.* Finally prove the property by model checking or theorem proving. In the example, all the formalised requirements were proved using both technologies except those that involve full number entry which could only be proved using theorem proving.

4 Developing a Model of the Device

The first step involved producing a model that could be analysed using model checking. This technology has the advantage that, since it is algorithmic, proof does not require a human prover. Theorem proving, on the other hand, usually requires proof guidance. The ingenuity in model checking is to formulate the properties appropriately and to interpret the results. The model under analysis had been developed in two parts. A generic "pump" component was developed that could be reused in other models. For example a BBraun infusion pump has also been studied in detail [8] and uses the same component. The Alaris version of the model focuses on mode behaviour. Proof with it is not tractable if the full number entry features of the model are also incorporated. To achieve tractability, token values were assumed for pump variables: vtbi, infusion rate, time and volume infused. They are taken to be integers in the range $0 \ldots 7$. These simplifications do not affect the mode behaviour of the device. The model used for the initial analysis was described in Modal Action Logic (MAL) [3] using the IVY tool [8]. MAL is a simple state transition language, easily translated from state transition diagrams or the SCR tabular format [9]. The notation is used because it is of a type that is more readily acceptable by developers. The MAL model is translated into NuSMV [5]. The properties that translate the requirements are expressed in CTL (see [6]). The following MAL modal axiom, involved in proving the requirement discussed in Sect. 7.1, describes conditions in which the button *key1* has the effect of confirming a device reset.

$$topline = clearsetup \rightarrow [key1]$$
$$topline' = holding \ \& \ middisp[drate]' \ \&$$
$$middisp[dvtbi]' \ \& \ !middisp[dtime]' \ \&$$
$$middisp[dvol]' \ \& \ !middisp[dbags]' \ \&$$
$$!middisp[dkvorate]' \ \& \ !middisp[dquery]' \ \&$$
$$fndisp1' = fvol \ \& \ fndisp2' = fvtbi \ \&$$
$$fndisp3' = fnull \ \& \ entrymode' = rmode \ \&$$
$$effect(device.reset) \ \& \ keep(bagscursor, rlock)$$

This axiom describes (to the right of [*key1*]) the effect of action *key1*. The expression to the left of the action (*topline = clearsetup*) states the condition under which the behaviour described for the action is performed. Hence, when the top line of the display shows "clear setup", and the action is invoked, then the expression on the right hand side describes the behaviour. Most of this behaviour changes the interface by defining values for attributes: *middisp, topline, fndisp1, fndisp2, fndisp3*. The priming of an attribute (for example, *topline'*) indicates that the action changes the value of that attribute. The action *key1* also changes the mode of the device (*entrymode*) to allow entry of infusion rate (*rmode*). It also invokes a generic pump action (*device.reset*) that initialises all the pump variables. This action *reset* is accessed in the reusable pump component which is identified as *device* in the MAL specification. The *keep*(...) expression specifies which attributes are not affected by the action and remain unchanged.

The MAL model focuses on interface features and the modes of the device, describing concretely how actions change the display and modes of the device. It has a simple discrete model of time. An action *tick* increments time as the infusion process continues, or while the device is paused. In the latter case the value of time is used to determine how long the pause has been. This model, even without full number entry, requires substantial processing for analysis – between one and two hours per property on a typical desktop computer.

A second model was developed by translating the MAL systematically into PVS [18] (a theorem proving system). The PVS specification allows the analysis in principle of properties involving infinitely many states. The equivalent specification for the fragment described above is:

```
key1_case_clearsetup(st: (per_key1)):alaris =
st WITH [ topline := holding,
          middisp := LAMBDA(x: imid_type):
            COND
              x = drate -> TRUE,
              x = dvtbi -> TRUE,
              x = dvol -> TRUE,
              x = dtime -> FALSE,
              x = dbags -> FALSE,
              x = dkvorate -> FALSE,
              x = dquery -> FALSE
            ENDCOND,
          device := reset(device(st)),
          fndisp1 := fvol, fndisp2 := fvtbi, fndisp3 := fnull,
          entrymode := rmode ]
```

The PVS theory captures all the characteristics of the MAL model, including time, but also includes a full number entry model. The PVS features that correspond to MAL elements can be clearly seen in the specification. This function key1_case_clearsetup is invoked in the more general key1 function when the condition topline(st) = clearsetup is true. The function has domain (per_key1) hence it is only permitted when key1 is accessible to the user. Note that the specification includes a set of predicates, of which per_key1 is an example, that are true if the action (in this case key1) is accessible to the user. The reason for having two models was that the counter-example approach supported by model checking facilitated analysis of the plausibility of the model and also refinement of the requirements in the early stages of development.

5   Validating the Model Against the Real Device

Plausibility was investigated first by checking properties and then by exploring the model through simulation [14]. A typical example of a property checked that, once relevant pump variables had been entered, infusion would lead to a state in which the volume infused was equal to the vtbi.

$$AG(device.infusionrate = 1 \ \& \ device.vtbi \ = \ 7 \rightarrow$$
$$AG(device.volumeinfused \ != \ 7))$$

Properties such as these are expressed as negations in order to construct a counter-example that has the required properties. This property asserts that it is always the case for all paths that if infusion rate is set to 1 (a token) and vtbi is set to 7 then a state cannot be reached in which volume infused is 7. This property does not depend on the details of the device user interface, depending only on the generic pump model, but produces results that enable an analysis of the interface, making possible a comparison between alternative interfaces. As expected, the property fails when checked and produces a trace of steps in which the infusion rate is set to 1 and vtbi is set to 7. It indicates that once this has happened, eventually the device is set to infuse, and then after more steps a state is reached where the volume that has been infused becomes 7. The trace can be compared with the actual device, thereby providing a visualisation of one possible path in the model.

The model checker (NuSMV [5]) accepts a finite state model and analyses it exhaustively to prove or disprove a property. Other model checkers that are not limited to finite state models do not significantly improve performance. They can complete the analysis in a reasonable time only if the models are not too large or complicated [7].

6   Formalising Requirements

Five FDA requirements described in [11] mitigate user related hazards:

R1. *Clearing the pump settings and resetting of the pump shall require confirmation.*
R2. *The pump shall issue an alert if paused for more than t minutes.*
R3. *If the pump is in a state where user input is required, the pump shall issue periodic alerts/indications every t minutes until the required input is provided.*
R4. *The flow rate for the pump shall be programmable.*
R5. *To avoid accidental tampering of the infusion pump's settings such as flow rate/vtbi, at least two steps should be required to change the setting.*
Further requirements were added based on templates supported by the IVY tool [8]. They mitigate various use or "interaction" hazards for infusion pumps identified in the hazard analysis presented in [16].
R6. *Whenever a pump variable is being entered, the variable should be clearly identified and its current value visible to the user.*

R7. *The current mode should be clearly identified. Changes in mode therefore should have perceivable feedback to that effect.*
R8. *Confirmation of number entry should be achieved using a consistent action.*
R9. *Any data entry action should be reversible.*

To prove the requirements of the model it is necessary to consider their *precise* interpretations. For reasons of space requirements R1, R2, R4 and R9 only will be considered. The formalisation uses a PVS like specification that combines a functional notation similar to that used in programming languages with logic connectives such as AND (conjunction), OR (disjunction), => (implication). Precision is achieved by defining abstractions that can be more readily understood and expressed as properties that can be proved of either the MAL or PVS models. The formalisation must capture the essence of the requirements as understood both by the regulator who developed it in the first place and the human factors specialists who can comment on the user aspects of the requirements and whether they are fulfilled by the specific properties of the device. The formalisation must not be biased towards a particular make of device.

6.1 R1: Clearing the Pump Settings and Resetting of the Pump Shall Require Confirmation

This requirement aims to prevent users changing infusion settings inadvertently. The state in which the particular pump variable is ready to clear is described by the predicate: `pumpvariable_ready_to_clear`. The `clear_setting` action for the device does not update the value until a `confirm_action` has taken place. Any other action (`no_confirm`), permitted by the device when `clear_setting` has occurred, has no effect on the pump variable if taken. Each pump setting is dealt with individually and, for pump variable vtbi, can be expressed as follows:

```
vtbi_ready_to_clear(st, x) AND x /= 0 =>
    (clear_setting_vtbi(st)'vtbi = x AND
    confirm_action(clear_setting(st))'vtbi = 0 AND
    no_confirm(clear_setting(st))'vtbi = x)
```

where: st is the current state of the device; vtbi is the state attribute that correspond to the considered pump variable; and x is the value of the considered pump variable before resetting.

6.2 R2: The Pump Shall Issue an Alert if Paused for More Than t Minutes

R2 requires that the user is alerted if the device is left unattended during data entry, as might occur if the clinician is interrupted. This requirement can be formulated as:

```
user_input_strictly_overdue(st) => alert(st)
```

where `user_input_strictly_overdue` is true if the device has been paused without activity for a specified period. This predicate can be expressed in more detail as:

```
user_input_strictly_overdue(st) = paused(st) AND
elapsed(st) > timeout
```

`paused` and `elapsed` will have specific meanings for the particular infusion pumps. `alert(st)` describes an appropriate alert produced by the device.

6.3   R4: The Flow Rate for the Pump Shall Be Programmable

This safety requirement ensures that any value for the flow rate can be programmed. The formalisation of the requirement indicates an inductive argument that proves there is always a sequence of actions to reach a particular value of the infusion rate. If the device is ready to enter the rate then there is always an action that will take the flow rate closer to the expected rate, and eventually the intended rate will be reached. For the illustrative purposes of the paper a simpler version of the requirement is adopted that demonstrates only that the flow rate gets closer to the expected rate (e) expressed as:

```
FORALL (st: State, e: infusion_rate):
rate_entry_ready(st) =>
     EXISTS (a: State -> State):
       (current_display_rate(st) > e =>
          (current_display_rate(st) - e >
                 current_display_rate(a(st)) - e))
       AND (current_display_rate(st) < e =>
                 (current_display_rate(st) - e <
                    current_display_rate(a(st)) - e))
```

The attribute `current_display_rate` is a visible representation of the current infusion rate.

6.4   R9: Any Data Entry Action Should Be Reversible

It seems desirable that for any number entry action there is an action that will reverse it. This can be expressed as:

```
ready_to_enter_pump_variable =>
FORALL (act1: State -> State): EXISTS (act2: State -> State):
        act2(act1(st))'pump_variable = st'pump_variable
```

This formulation reveals interesting features of many of the number entry schemes for infusion pumps, because, as discussed below, in general this simple notion of reversibility is not possible.

7   Proving Requirements

Theorem proving uses natural deduction to do proof. Induction can be used to prove general properties over very large numbers of states. For this reason properties can be proved that are beyond the capacity of readily available computers using model checking. Setting up the induction and guiding the proof requires skill. When a proof fails it can be difficult to see why it has gone wrong and what must be done to remedy it — a process that is relatively straightforward using a model checker through available counter-examples.

Proof by model checking provides clear counter-examples that aid diagnosis and reformulation of models and properties. Proof by theorem proving is faster but failure requires more skill to interpret. In the present case the two safety requirements (R4 and R9), that require precise modelling of the number entry system of the device, could not be proved using model checking. R1 and R2 could be proved using both model checking and theorem proving. Model checking required approximately 90 min using an Intel 2.4 GHz i5 with 8 GB of RAM (1333 MHz DDR3) when the properties are taken individually.

The first stage in proving a requirement is to take the formalisations discussed in Sect. 6 and to further refine them as properties of the particular device.

7.1   Proving R1: Clearing the Pump Settings and Resetting of the Pump Shall Require Confirmation

The Alaris device is ready to clear vtbi when the device is powered on and in the holding state. The pump variable needs clearing so should be non-zero. Relevant state attributes for expressing whether the pump is infusing and switched on are infusing? and powered_on. The vtbi_ready_to_clear predicate is therefore:

```
vtbi_ready_to_clear(st: alaris, x: ivols): bool =
NOT device(st)'infusing? AND device(st)'powered_on? AND
device(st)'vtbi=x AND x \= 0
```

clear_setting(st: alaris): alaris = on(on(st)) because *on* switches the device off if switched on and vice versa. clear_user_confirm(st: alaris): alaris = key1(st). That key3 is the only other available action is checked by the predicate no_confirm that specifies that the chevron keys, key2, query, run and pause are not available:

```
no_confirm(st: alaris): boolean =
NOT (per_sup(st) OR per_fup(st) OR per_sdown(st) OR per_fdown(st)
OR per_key2(st) OR per_query(st) OR per_run(st) OR per_pause(st))
```

The theorem combines these elements:

```
R1vtbi: THEOREM
FORALL (st: alaris, x: ivols):
LET stprime=clear_setting(st) IN (vtbi_ready_to_clear(st,x) =>
```

```
(topline(stprime) = clearsetup AND device(stprime)'vtbi=x
AND no_confirm(stprime) AND device(key1(stprime))'vtbi=0
AND device(key3(stprime))'vtbi=x))
```

The assertion captured in the theorem is required to be proved of all states and is easy to prove in PVS. The general purpose proof command **grind** proves the theorem. In most other theorems it is necessary to restrict the proof to reachable states. This must be done explicitly when theorem proving, but is checked automatically by the model checker.

7.2 Proving R2: The Pump Shall Issue an Alert if Paused for More Than t Minutes

The user_input_strictly_overdue predicate is defined as:

```
user_input_strictly_overdue(st: alaris): bool =
   device(st)'powered_on? AND NOT device(st)'infusing? AND
     (device(st)'elapse > timeout)
```

The attribute elapse specifies the time since the device was last used when in holding mode. elapse is incremented when the device is paused each time the tick action is invoked. The alert is specified as: alert(st: alaris): boolean = topline(st) = attention. An assumption is that the alert is only indicated by an appropriate top line on the display. In practice there is also an audible alarm. These additional features are easily modelled. The assertion that is to be proved refines the property of Sect. 6.2 as follows.

```
R2assertionwithouttick(st: alaris): boolean =
      user_input_strictly_overdue(st) => alert(st)
```

The theorem is formulated as a structural induction. It requires that, over all states that can be reached from the initial state by an Alaris action, the assertion is true. The predicate alaris_transitions expresses this reachability property:

```
alaris_transitions
(pre, post: alaris): boolean =
(per_sup(pre) & post = sup(pre)) OR (per_fup(pre) & post = fup(pre)) OR
(per_sdown(pre) & post = sdown(pre)) OR
(per_fdown(pre) & post = fdown(pre)) OR
(per_tick(pre) & post = tick(pre)) OR (per_key1(pre) & post = key1(pre)) OR
(per_key2(pre) & post = key2(pre)) OR (per_key3(pre) & post = key3(pre)) OR
(per_query(pre) & post = query(pre)) OR post = on(pre) OR
(per_run(pre) & post = run(pre)) OR (per_pause(pre) & post = pause(pre))
```

The state **pre** is associated with the state **post** by an action that is permitted by the device. The appropriate permission predicate is omitted when the action is always permitted. The theorem that uses the structural induction is as follows.

```
R2withouttick: THEOREM
FORALL (pre, post: alaris):
(init?(pre) => R2assertionwithouttick(pre)) AND
((R2assertionwithouttick(pre) AND
alaris_transitions(pre, post)) => R2assertionwithouttick(post))
```

7.3 Proving R4: The Flow Rate for the Pump Shall Be Programmable

The components required in the formalisation are as follows.

```
rate_entry_ready(st: alaris): boolean =
switchedon?(st) AND NOT rlock(st) AND
(((entrymode(st) = rmode) AND (topline(st) = holding)) OR
((entrymode(st) = infusemode) AND (topline(st) = infusing)))
```

The device is ready to accept a rate value when: the device is switched on; infusion rate is not locked; and the top line shows holding or infusing. Further redundant constraints are included, relating to entry mode, to focus the states under consideration in the proof.

Two possible actions are dealt with in the theorem. If the expected rate exceeds the current display rate, then the single chevron up key moves the current display rate closer to the expected rate. On the other hand if the current display rate exceeds the expected rate, the single chevron down will get the current display rate closer. This theorem could be extended by using the size of the difference to use double or single chevron keys. However a simpler version is adopted that nevertheless fulfils the requirement. The current display rate is defined for the Alaris as: `current_display_rate(st: alaris): irates = device(st)'infusionrate` The theorem is based on the formulation of Sect. 6.3.

```
R4: THEOREM
FORALL (st: alaris, expected_rate: irates):
(rate_entry_ready(st) =>
    (((expected_rate > current_display_rate(st)
AND per_sup(st) =>
    (expected_rate - current_display_rate(sup(st))) <
    (expected_rate - current_display_rate(st)))) AND
    ((expected_rate < current_display_rate(st)
AND per_sdown(st) =>
    (current_display_rate(sdown(st)) - expected_rate) <
    (current_display_rate(st) - expected_rate)))))
```

An element of the theorem, not expressed in the formulation of Sect. 6.3, checks that the action is available to the user before applying it.

7.4   Proving R9: Any Data Entry Action Should Be Reversible

Reversibility of number entry actions is only satisfied by the device in limited situations. For example:

- Applying double chevron up to 99 and then applying double chevron down produces 90.
- Applying double chevron down to 100 and then applying double chevron up produces 91.
- Applying single chevron up to 99.9 and then applying single chevron down produces 99.
- Applying single chevron down to 100 and then applying single chevron up produces 99.9.

These anomalies arise because there are thresholds in which the effect of the chevron action changes. The effect of the action depends on the current value within that threshold. Hence because 99.9 is less than 100 single chevron up increments by 0.1. But now it is greater than or equal to 100, so single chevron down decrements by 1. These anomalies were "discovered" through a process of trial and error, successively reformulating the theorem until it was proved true. One of the several theorems proved in this category, which elaborates the formulation of Sect. 6.4, is:

```
R9ratesdownsupqpt1: THEOREM
FORALL (st: alaris):
 (rate_entry_ready(st) AND
 per_sup(st) AND per_sdown(release_sup(sup(st))) AND
 (device(st)'infusionrate >= 0) AND
 ((device(st)'infusionrate + small_step/10) <100) AND
 (floor(device(st)'infusionrate*10) =
         device(st)'infusionrate*10) AND
 (ceil_rate(device(st)'infusionrate*10) =
  device(st)'infusionrate*10)) =>
   device(release_sdown(sdown(release_sup(sup(st)))))'infusionrate
                        = device(st)'infusionrate)
```

rate_entry_ready is as specified in the case of R4 and small_step is defined to be 1. Further clauses in the theorem are concerned with (1) affirming that the appropriate number entry action is available to the user; (2) specifying that the number is expressed with no greater precision than one decimal place and (3) including the release action that is required after pressing any chevron button to indicate that the button has been released (note that any chevron button can be held down, thereby increasing the size of the increment or decrement achieved by the button). This theorem is true for all states without the need for induction. However constraint of the numbers to one decimal place is required in the proof. This is a property of the number entry system on the Alaris that should be proved and would require a structural induction to prove it. Similar parts of the theorem have been proved for the ranges 100 to 1000 and greater than 1000.

Proof of the last requirement, with all its qualifications, is of little value as an assurance that number entry actions are easily reversible by users. The qualifications that were developed in attempting to prove the theorem were however valuable in understanding the characteristics of the number entry system. Indeed formulating and proving the theorem raises questions as to whether the device is acceptable or whether it is likely to lead to interaction error. It should be noted that the latest release of Alaris firmware has fixed these inconsistencies.

8 Discussion and Conclusions

Demonstrating that the design of a medical device has been constructed to reduce the probability of interaction error to "as low as reasonably practicable" is a serious issue. It is estimated that there were 56,000 adverse event reports relating to infusion pumps between 2005 to 2009 in the United States including at least 500 deaths. This has resulted in 87 infusion pump recalls to address identified safety concerns, according to FDA data. Of these adverse event reports interaction error has been a significant factor. The documentation provided by manufacturers to regulators as part of a safety argument is usually substantial. However, the scale of the argument inevitably makes it difficult for regulators to comprehend them and to be confident that the evidence provided is of satisfactory quality. The use of formal techniques has a number of potential advantages. (1) It is precise and concise. (2) Tools like model checkers and theorem provers provided to support them enable mechanical and exhaustive verification. (3) The use of simulation techniques combined with the specification can clearly demonstrate how potential problems are addressed.

There are however obstacles to the immediate take-up of these facilities. They are not currently part of a typical developer's suite of tools. They are not currently used in product development. However there are signs of interest in these techniques. For example the FDA has developed generic PCA models [17] using Simulink. It is not however a feasible option to expect regulators to construct models after the fact. An ideal option would be that manufacturers produce models as part of their design process demonstrating that a submitted product adheres to safety requirements. The regulators would then use tools to validate the models provided as part of the developer's submission.

In the present study model checking of properties combined with simulation was used to support the process of validation of models by generating traces to be validated on the device. However, manufacturers have access to source code and even if they don't develop their devices using models they can create faithful models systematically. A further important issue not addressed here is how to validate that the considered set of safety requirements correctly address the usability and safety of the device for the context in which the device is to be used. This problem is orthogonal to the techniques presented in this paper. Safety aspects can be addressed with a human factors emphasis using a hazard analysis such as the one presented in [14].

This paper has described one experience using formal verification technologies to verify draft FDA safety requirements for a commercial medical device. Examples were illustrated in detail to explore three key verification challenges: how to validate a model and show that it is a faithful representation of the device; the benefits of formalising requirements given in natural language; how to prove requirements on realistic models of devices. Our main contribution is to demonstrate how to achieve the FDA's agenda of using formal methods that can support the approval process for real medical devices. In particular requirements related to interaction issues have been formalised and verified.

Formalising the requirements provides benefits in addition to the ability to prove them. It led to much more detailed thinking about the precise nature of the requirements, both in general and for a specific device, than was possible in the informal natural language version. The pragmatic and informal combination of model checking and theorem proving provided powerful tools for analysis. By using each flexibly for requirements they were suited to, rather than ideologically favouring one for all requirements, or trying to combine them into a single tool applying both, it was possible to prove the requirements with minimum effort. One potential drawback of this approach is the need to master the two verification techniques. Indeed, both verification methods currently require significant skills for analysis. However, we have observed recurrent patterns in the structure of the formal models of devices from different manufacturers, and in the strategies needed to complete verification of several types of safety requirements. Therefore there are clear opportunities to create a reference template that can be used to automate the approach and thus reduce the analysis effort.

Acknowledgements. This work has been funded by the EPSRC research grant EP/G059063/1: CHI+MED (Computer–Human Interaction for Medical Devices). J.C. Campos was funded by project NORTE-07-0124-FEDER-000062. We thank our reviewers for valuable and constructive feedback.

References

1. Abrial, J.-R.: Modeling in Event-B: System and Software Engineering. Cambridge University Press, Cambridge (2010)
2. Arney, D., Jetley, R., Jones, P., Lee, I., Sokolsky, O., Ray, A., Zhang, Y.: Generic infusion pump hazard analysis and safety requirements. Technical report MS-CIS-08-31, University of Pennsylvania, February 2009
3. Campos, J.C., Harrison, M.D.: Interaction engineering using the IVY tool. In: Calvary, G., Graham, T.C.N., Gray, P. (eds.) Proceedings of the ACM SIGCHI Symposium on Engineering Interactive Computing Systems, pp. 35–44. ACM Press (2009)
4. Cardinal Health Inc.: Alaris GP volumetric pump: directions for use. Technical report, Cardinal Health, 1180 Rolle, Switzerland (2006)
5. Cimatti, A., et al.: NuSMV 2: an opensource tool for symbolic model checking. In: Brinksma, E., Larsen, K.G. (eds.) CAV 2002. LNCS, vol. 2404, pp. 359–364. Springer, Heidelberg (2002). doi:10.1007/3-540-45657-0_29

6. Clarke, E.M., Grumberg, O., Peled, D.A.: Model Checking. MIT Press, Cambridge (1999)
7. Gelman, G.E., Feigh, K.M., Rushby, J.: Example of a complementary use of model checking and agent-based simulation. In: 2013 IEEE International Conference on Systems, Man, and Cybernetics (SMC), pp. 900–905, October 2013
8. Harrison, M.D., Campos, J.C., Masci, P.: Reusing models and properties in the analysis of similar interactive devices. In: Innovations in Systems and Software Engineering, pp. 1–17, April 2013
9. Heitmeyer, J.C., Kirby Jr., J., Labaw, B.: Applying the SRC requirements method to a weapons control panel: an experience report. In: Proceedings of the Second Workshop on Formal Methods in Software Practice (FMSP 1998), pp. 92–102 (1998)
10. Holzmann, G.J.: Trends in software verification. In: Araki, K., Gnesi, S., Mandrioli, D. (eds.) FME 2003. LNCS, vol. 2805, pp. 40–50. Springer, Heidelberg (2003). doi:10.1007/978-3-540-45236-2_4
11. Jetley, R., Purushothaman Iyer, S., Jones, P.L.: A formal methods approach to medical device review. Computer **39**(4), 61–67 (2006)
12. Leveson, N.G.: Engineering a Safer World: Systems Thinking Applied to Safety (Engineering Systems). MIT Press, Cambridge (2011)
13. Masci, P., Ayoub, A., Curzon, P., Harrison, M.D., Lee, I., Sokolsky, O., Thimbleby, H.: Verification of interactive software for medical devices: PCA infusion pumps and FDA regulation as an example. In: Proceedings ACM Symposium Engineering Interactive Systems (EICS 2013), pp. 81–90. ACM Press (2013)
14. Masci, P., Ayoub, A., Curzon, P., Lee, I., Sokolsky, O., Thimbleby, H.: Model-based development of the generic PCA infusion pump user interface prototype in PVS. In: Bitsch, F., Guiochet, J., Kaâniche, M. (eds.) SAFECOMP 2013. LNCS, vol. 8153, pp. 228–240. Springer, Heidelberg (2013). doi:10.1007/978-3-642-40793-2_21
15. Masci, P., Zhang, Y., Jones, P., Curzon, P., Thimbleby, H.: Formal Verification of Medical Device User Interfaces Using PVS. In: Gnesi, S., Rensink, A. (eds.) FASE 2014. LNCS, vol. 8411, pp. 200–214. Springer, Heidelberg (2014). doi:10.1007/978-3-642-54804-8_14
16. Masci, P., Zhang, Y., Jones, P., Thimbleby, H., Curzon, P.: A generic user interface architecture for analyzing use hazards in infusion pump software. In: Turau, V., Kwiatkowska, M., Mangharam, R., Weyer, C. (eds.) 5th Workshop on Medical Cyber-Physical Systems. OpenAccess Series in Informatics (OASIcs), vol. 36, pp. 1–14. Schloss Dagstuhl-Leibniz-Zentrum fuer Informatik, Dagstuhl (2014)
17. Murugesan, A., Whalen, M.W., Rayadurgam, S., Heimdahl, M.P.E.: Compositional verification of a medical device system. In: Proceedings ACM High Integrity Language Technologies (HILT 2013). ACM Press (2013)
18. Owre, S., Rushby, J.M., Shankar, N.: PVS: a prototype verification system. In: Kapur, D. (ed.) CADE 1992. LNCS, vol. 607, pp. 748–752. Springer, Heidelberg (1992). doi:10.1007/3-540-55602-8_217
19. US Food and Drug Administration: General principles of software validation; final guidance for industry and FDA staff. Technical report, Center for Devices and Radiological Health, January 2002. http://www.fda.gov/medicaldevices/deviceregulationandguidance

Secure and Customizable EHR Management Services with COASTmed

Alegria Baquero$^{(\boxtimes)}$ and Richard N. Taylor

Institute for Software Research, University of California, Irvine, USA
{abaquero,taylor}@ics.uci.edu

Abstract. The exchange of electronic health records (EHR) among multiple parties and for multiple purposes raises nontrivial concerns. Unfortunately, privacy and operational policies granting individual access privileges to parties are often artifacts foreign to healthcare systems, thus EHR security is all the more frail. Moreover, current web service technologies that constitute many EHR systems treat users uniformly, making it more difficult for information consumers to use this data for specific purposes. Therefore, there is a need for EHR systems that offer secure, policy compliant access to data services and enable users to obtain the required information according to their individual authority. We present COASTmed, a notional EHR system that simultaneously offers provider-controlled differential service access and user-controlled customization. Our prototype is founded on the architectural principles of the COAST style and leverages the Rei policy language.

Keywords: Computational web services · Decentralization · Policies · Healthcare

1 Introduction

Healthcare is largely a decentralized enterprise—a network of people and organizations are involved in some aspect of patients' healthcare, constantly accessing and sharing patient information. A nontrivial consequence of these interactions, which raises privacy concerns, is the dispersion of patient data among uncountable (even unknown) physical and digital locations. Despite HIPAA regulations and other locally imposed privacy and operational policies to protect patients' data, there are precedents of privacy breaches due to, for example, insiders' authority abuse [1]. The preeminent problem is that these policies are isolated from information systems' operations and therefore services for users within and foreign to an organization do not always comply with these regulations.

A second, no less important problem is that patient information is used for diverse (often unanticipated) purposes. Yet, it is unfeasible for information service providers—namely organizations holding patient data—to deliver personalized information for every current and future user and need. Although Web service technologies are being deployed to deliver patient information in

© Springer International Publishing AG 2017
M. Huhn and L. Williams (Eds.): FHIES 2014/SEHC 2014, LNCS 9062, pp. 129–144, 2017.
DOI: 10.1007/978-3-319-63194-3_9

replacement of the exchange of physical documents, these are rigid, unilaterally controlled "one-size-fits-all" solutions with a "minimum common denominator" set of capabilities. These services, hardly satisfy any of their users' needs and curtail access rights to otherwise more privileged users.

Given these problems, there is a need for information services more suitable for this complex domain involving an intricate network of users and uses of patient data, heterogenous trust relationships among parties, and convoluted legal and privacy strictures. We identify two salient challenges of these novel information services: (a) granting access to patient data according to appropriate, desired relationships between individuals and organizations, and; (b) allow authorized information users to obtain the required patient data for diverse uses.

Our goals are twofold. First, enabling differential access to a information provider's services, where the provider can distinguish among service consumers, making available patient data and computational capability according to formally defined privacy and operational policies. Differential service provision allows organizations to treat users idiosyncratically, maintaining multiple trust relationships, and deliberately restricting and expanding the per-user availability of data and functionality. An information service provider may be, for example, a healthcare provider, an insurance company, a government agency, and so on. Second, enabling service customization so that service consumers can use patient information and computational capabilities at will, however within individual authority and access rights. Service users or consumers, in the context of web services, are other software components or systems within or external to an organization. In short, we provide EHR information and management services which are offered according to rigorous privacy and operational policies and which can be customized by the user to the extent of their authority.

Key insights lead to our solution fulfilling these goals. First, given that trust is crucial for data disclosure, it is necessary to clearly capture trust relationships to support access control mechanisms. Second, considering decentralization is essential—autonomous parties act according to individual interests and critical data constantly crosses organizations' boundaries. Third, security needs to be inherent to any solution, and not bolted-on after the fact. Fourth, given the complex legal and ethical regulations involved, information services ought to be tightly coupled with and behave according to established policies. Lastly, given the difficulty of provider-controlled service personalization to an increasing number of users, the burden of customization needs to lie on data consumers.

Our solution consists on (a) combining formal policies and the architectural principles and techniques of the COAST architectural style [2] for achieving fine-grained customization and policy-based differential access to patient information and computational services, and; (b) assessing the suitability and feasibility of the proposed techniques through conceptual and technical analyses and the development of COASTmed, a notional EHR system offering services through these novel techniques. The outcome of this work are novel techniques to protect patient data services while allowing parties to manipulate and make meaningful use of the information they are authorized to access.

Our work approaches the essential need of speedy and safe exchange of distributed patient data in support of efficient and coordinated healthcare delivery, epidemic outbreak surveillance, health sciences research, and other socially beneficial goals. Our context is decentralized information systems, whose constituent services operate under multiple authorities. This work is relevant within Service Oriented Architectures, yet our approach is fundamentally different from current uniform, rigid, and unilaterally provided Web services—COASTmed's services are computationally enabled, customizable, and user-specific, exposing patient data and system capabilities according to formal policies. Our work applies access control features—providers define per-user authority over their services—and it is further motivated by the insufficiency of traditional access control models for complex, large-scale decentralized domains such as federated healthcare [3]. Our work on secure and customizable healthcare data services is rooted on the principles of the COAST architectural style [2], which succeeds current Web architectures to meet increasing openness, flexibility, dynamicity, and security demands. We also build on privacy and policy languages by formalizing organizational policies describing data disclosure and service access conditions.

In the next section we set forth the architectural foundations of COASTmed, describe a set of motivating scenarios, and detail the system's design (Sect. 2). In Sect. 3, we provide a comparative evaluation of COASTmed and other healthcare technologies with comparable goals. Finally, we discuss our evaluation results (Sect. 4) and present conclusions and plans for future work (Sect. 5).

2   COASTmed

The goal of COASTmed is to provide diverse parties customized access and use of electronic health record data according to their individual authority. COASTmed is rooted in architectural principles involving capability-based security and computation exchange, along with formal policy specifications to enable policy-based differential access to customizable EHR information services.

2.1   Motivating Scenarios

The following scenarios address shortcomings in the domain regarding the lack of immediately available data, systems and services policy compliance, patient information privacy and security, the invariability and inflexibility of information services, and the integration of distributed and independently managed data.

John accesses an online service to make an appointment with Dr. Smith. At the time of the appointment, John uses a mobile user interface assistant to send a single-use Capability URL (CURL) [4]—a reference to a service with authority semantics—to the doctor's computer to allow her to access, on the spot, a laboratory's service to obtain John's blood work results. The issued CURL is created by the lab according to its own privacy policies upon the patient's request. Dr. Smith can only access the most recent results and the CURL can never be used again. These restrictions are implicitly embedded in the CURL to preserve the patient's privacy. The doctor then sends a custom algorithm to the lab's service, using the issued CURL, to perform specialized data analyses and diagnostics.

Jane has been diagnosed with hip osteoarthritis and requires a hip replacement. Concerned about the expenses, Jane uses a CURL issued by her physician to access her health record where the recommended procedures are recorded. She sends a custom computation with the procedure's code to her insurance company's service by way of a policy-holder-specific CURL. The service identifies the patient through metadata encoded within the incoming CURL. The custom computation executes, calculating the expected expenses based on her insurance plan. Her insurance company also allows Jane to compare the costs of various providers in the area using a patient-specific service.

Researchers are investigating the relationship between diabetes and cardiovascular diseases. Multiple healthcare providers, according to their own privacy policies, issue a CURL for the researchers use. The capabilities conferred by CURLs restrict the access to specific patients' records, but enable the researchers to retrieve aggregate patient data and compose custom statistical algorithms with the functions within the authorized binding environment. Healthcare institutions offer similar services to pharmaceutical companies for the evaluation of prescription drugs through periodic analyses of patients' treatment and outcomes. Similarly, the CDC installs long-running computations within peers of key healthcare facilities to detect epidemic outbreaks. Healthcare providers generate and distribute CURLs addressing policy-conforming, privacy-aware, and specialized services which provide the degree and depth of access parties have agreed upon, limiting functional capability to specific needs.

2.2   Architectural Foundations

The architecture of a software system involves the overarching design decisions governing its behavior. Our approach to secure and custom services is founded on the COmputAtional State Transfer (COAST) architectural style [2] and the expressiveness of the Rei policy language [5].

COAST subsumes content under the bilateral computational exchange among autonomous and decentralized peers. COAST provides a set of design principles for building decentralized, secure, and highly adaptive systems. In COAST:

- all services are computations whose sole means of interaction is the asynchronous messaging of primitive data types, data structures, closures, continuations, and binding environments (map of key/value pairs);
- a computation is the execution of a closure c by execution engine ϵ within the lexical context of binding environment β, therefore all computations execute within the confines of some execution site $\langle \epsilon, \beta \rangle$;
- computations are named by capability URLs (CURLs), unforgeable, cryptographic structures that convey the authority to communicate (x may deliver a message to y only if x holds a CURL u_y of y).

In COAST, application state is driven by message exchange; control and data flows among computations, thus state progresses by way of decentralized collaboration. COAST has strong emphasis on decentralization, a crucial property of the healthcare domain. Its foundations in mobility and the ability to compose closures from bindings provided by computations affords a customization power not achievable with current Web services. COAST is designed to provide on-demand services which are created and terminated independently. In addition, the autonomy of computations promotes system scalability through the independent creation and evolution of services.

COAST provides built-in security through the Principle of Least Authority by which users are only granted the privileges necessary to complete their task. Moreover, COAST's capability-based security is enabled through cryptographically signed CURLs which confer authority and rights to communicate with another computation. A CURL u_x implicitly denotes the services offered by x, bestowing functional capability to closures sent in messages to x using u_x. Therefore, capability-based security permits providing differential access to services to distinct users. Computations run within bounded execution environments, mitigating the threats characteristic of mobile code. In addition, islands are self-certified and communication between computations is encrypted.

Although architectural styles are detached from implementation details, the Motile/Island infrastructure is provided to assist in the development of COAST applications. Motile is a language for the serialization and exchange of mobile code among COAST peers. Islands are the implementation of peers—single address spaces defined by an IP address/port combination—which host actors, the reification of COAST computations.

We have chosen to found our studies in COAST given that its emphasis on security, decentralization, and dynamicity are appropriate and necessary to cope with changing trust relationships in the healthcare domain.

Rei is a logic-based policy language in which policies are expressed in terms of rights, prohibitions, obligations, and dispensations. Although Rei is domain independent, policy specification relies on domain vocabularies.

Policies are rules associated to subjects. A Rei policy is formally represented as *has(Subject, PolicyObject)* where *subject* is a class or entity (e.g., physician, Dr. Smith). A *PolicyObject* is either a *right, obligation, prohibition,* or *dispensation,* described as *PolicyObject(Action, Conditions)*. For example, the policy "a subject has the right to print if he/she is an employee" is expressed *has(Person, right (printAction, (employee (Person))))*. Moreover, an action can be more articulately described as *action(ActionName, TargetObjects, Pre-Conditions, Effects)*. Rei also provides syntax to express action order and cardinality: *seq(A,B)* (A then B), *nond(A,B)* (A or B), *repetition(A)*, and *once(A)*; and express complex conditions using the logical conjunctions *and* and *or*, and negation *not*.

Rei was chosen among other policy languages after thorough evaluations due to its compact, well-defined, and expressive logic-based syntax for describing healthcare policies, as well as its natural compatibility with COAST.

2.3 System Design

At startup, the root computation at a healthcare provider's COAST island creates a set of computations to (a) manage domain ontologies; (b) manage and evaluate policies; (c) associate policies with system capabilities; (d) generate user-specific service CURLs, and; (e) create user-specific services.

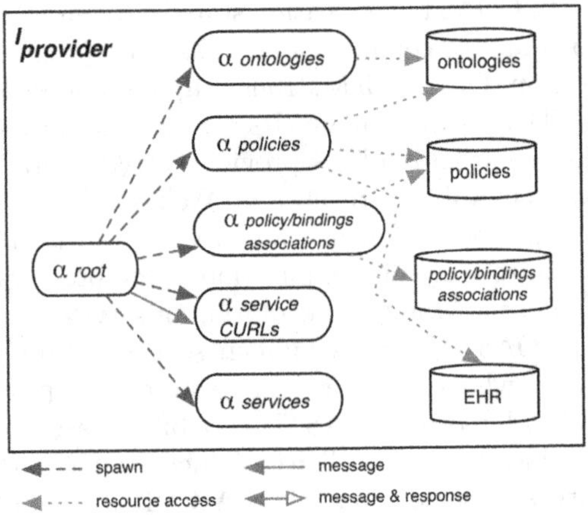

Fig. 1. The initial system architecture of a healthcare provider's COAST island

Policy Specification. Privacy-aware services provide patient data solely to authorized parties with distinct access privileges. To guide the behavior of services, it is necessary to capture organizational policies which describe the conditions under which data is disclosed. COASTmed allows formalizing privacy and operational policies through a constrained version of the Rei policy language. For example, a policy which states that only cardiologists are allowed to access the portion of medical records pertinent to cardiac ailments may be specified as:

```
policy(Physician,right(action(access,(cardiac_ehrs)),(
    instanceOf(Physician,cardiologist)))))
```

Policies bestow rights according to zero or more conditions. In the previous policy, the condition `instanceOf(Physician,cardiologist)` requires the subject in the physician role to be a cardiologist. Policies can refer abstractly to subjects and objects by referring to roles and object categories. These are capitalized in formal policies and implemented as variables. For example, in the previous policy, `Physician` refers to a principal's role. However, our approach is not limited to roles, but to specific principals. For instance, the previous abstract policy can be specific to a particular physician by replacing `Physician` with `drJones`.

Policy specification can include domain vocabularies to increase shared understanding of policies within healthcare organizations. For example, the policy:

```
policy(Physician,right(action(prescribe(fluoroquinolones),
    Patient),(diagnosis(Patient,anthrax)))))
```

states that a physician can prescribe fluoroquinolones if the patient has been diagnosed with anthrax. Both *fluoroquinolones* and *anthrax* are domain terms within the ATC code and the ICD-10 ontologies correspondingly.

COASTmed's architecture includes a specialized computation *αpolicies* (where α stands for *actor*, a computation's implementation model) which allows creating, modifying and evaluating policies (Fig. 1). Evaluation of abstract policies, thus those containing capitalized variables, require real data to replace those variables. At an incoming request for service, COASTmed retrieves from the database the set of roles that the principal fulfills within the organization and filters out the policies that are not relevant to these roles. Then, policy variables are replaced with constants (e.g., `Physician` is replaced by the principal's name) and each condition (i.e. predicate) is evaluated against facts within the database to obtain a truth value. Specific principal rights described within policies are granted when all its predicates evaluate to true.

Service Definitions. A COAST island is initialized with a set on initial capabilities or functions. For instance, a healthcare provider's island has functions to create, modify, and share electronic health records, register personnel within roles, create and evaluate policies, and so on. A root computation can jumpstart a number of computations or services with diverse capabilities or *spawn* new services as a result of incoming messages. As previously described, a service is a computation executed in the context of a binding environment. Binding environments are the set of primitive values, data structures, and functions existing within the service's scope and which are made available to consumers.

As shown in Fig. 1, the root computation spawns the services *αontologies*, *αpolicies*, *αpolicy/bindings-associations*, *αservice-CURLs*, and *αservices*, each with their own capabilities. For example, *αpolicies* includes functions such as `policies/create` and `policies/evaluate` within its binding environment. User-specific services thus include a subset of the root's capabilities, which are assigned according to privacy and operational policies.

Policy and Service Bindings. Differential, user-specific services are provided to patients, doctors, nurses, insurance companies, and other domain participants according to organizational policies. For doing so, COASTmed enables associating policies with island bindings. For example, a policy stating that a principal has the right to create electronic health records if he/she is a physician

```
policy(Person,right(action(create,(ehr)),(instanceOf(Person,
    physician)))))
```

is associated with the function `ehr/create`, association stored within a database. Therefore, if all the policy's predicates evaluate to true, then the principal or subject is authorized to use the `ehr/create` function; this function will be made available within the user-specific service binding environment.

Service CURLs and Dynamic Service Creation. As described, a healthcare provider evaluates the policies whose subject match the roles or the identity of a first-time service user. The authorized binding environment for that user is then the set of functions that are associated with the policies that evaluate to *true*. Following, the *αservice-CURLs* computation (Fig. 1) generates and returns a user-specific CURL addressing *αservices*. Recall that CURLs are

COAST's mechanisms to address and send messages to services or computations. Since a CURL can embed arbitrary data as metadata, the names of the authorized bindings or binding environments are embedded within the generated CURL. CURLs are tamper-proof, therefore it is not possible for a malicious party to expand its authority to healthcare providers' services.

When the consumer uses the issued CURL (which addresses $\alpha services$) to access the authorized service, $\alpha services$ retrieves the information regarding the authorized bindings from the CURL's metadata and dynamically creates, within an independent thread of execution, a new user-specific service whose lexical scope is limited those bindings—the user has only those functionalities available and nothing else. The user's message is forwarded to this newly created, personalized service for evaluation. If a custom closure exist within the message, it will execute only if it is composed by the authorized bindings; otherwise, the message will be rejected if it attempts to use a function that is not within this bounded execution context (even if the function exists within the island).

User-specific services are created dynamically for efficiency and scalability given that users, such as patients, may use the service sporadically. Constantly executing user services misuses resources (i.e. memory and processing power).

Using and Customizing Services. Service consumers use COAST-enabled services through issued CURLs. A message may contain primitive values, data structures, or custom closures that leverage the user-specific authorized bindings. As described, $\alpha services$ inspects the CURL's metadata for information regarding the authorized system capabilities for that user and dynamically creates a bounded service in which to evaluate the incoming message. Issued CURLs have an expiration date and may also have a limited use count for security and increased control over a principal's privileges. For instance, a user can continue using the service as long as a CURL is not expired, has a use count greater than zero, and has not been revoked by the service provider.

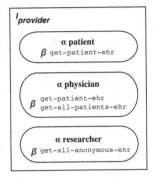

Fig. 2. A COAST peer running 3 user services

Not only can the bindings provided by services be used "as is", but customization can be achieved through functional composition using the authorized bindings. In other words, given that actors themselves are computational environments, the available bindings within an actor can be combined to compose custom closures. For example, a COAST peer may have, at startup, three services running (Fig. 2): one for John ($\alpha patient$), another for Dr. Smith ($\alpha physician$), and a third one for Dr. Jones ($\alpha researcher$), each with their binding environment (denoted by β)[1]. Dr. Jones, using a CURL @researcher sends $\alpha researcher$, for example, a custom closure $\lambda average\text{-}age$:

---

[1] Figure 2 illustrates a partial view of the system, depicting only the service provider.

(lambda() (....(get-all-anonymous-ehr)....)) which leverages the available get-all-anonymous-ehr function to compute the average age of patients with diabetes. Hence, although the function to obtain the desired data was not explicitly provided by the service, COAST allows customizing services by way of function composition and code mobility.

Differential Service Provision is enabled through policy bounded capabilities which are selectively included within user-specific binding environments and are addressed by CURLs. Figure 2 illustrates an island $I_{provider}$ with functions get-patient-ehr, get-all-patients-ehr, and get-all-anonymous-ehr, where three different user services are assigned one or more island's capabilities. If, for example, John, a patient who only has a CURL @patient for service $\alpha patient$, sends a custom closure that includes the function get-all-patients-ehr, the message will be discarded since get-all-patients-ehr does not exist within $\alpha patient$'s binding environment ($\beta patient$). Figure 3 shows a sequence where a service consumer issues a service request and receives a CURL to communicate with the authorized user-specific service; following the user uses the service by sending a message with a custom closure using the service's CURL.

Service Evolution. Services evolve for reasons such as the availability of new capabilities, changes in privacy and operational policies, or to purposely expand or constrain principals' services. Service evolution mainly involves the modification of binding environments assigned to user services, affecting also their CURLs' metadata. When policies change, some or all users may be affected; their user CURLs are revoked, therefore no longer usable, and new ones are issued to users.

COASTmed Prototype. We have built the COASTmed EHR prototype using COAST's Motile/Island infrastructure [2]. COASTmed currently allows a remote

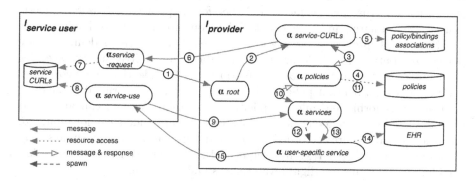

Fig. 3. A service consumer's service request and use

policy maker to specify Rei-based policies, integrated with functions that allow obtaining, for the purpose of evaluation, data from a patient database. At a user's request for service, CURLs are generated based on the user's identity, the result of the evaluation of policies relevant to the user's identity and role, and the associations of policies and island capabilities. Moreover, new COAST services with the authorized binding environments are created to evaluate users' messages received via the issued CURLs. The prototype is deployed on a single Linux machine; at startup several COAST islands (distinct ip addresses/port pairs) are created for different stakeholders (e.g., healthcare provider, policy maker, physician, and so on). This prototype allows us to simulate scenarios of authorized and customizable information access and capability use.

3 Comparative Evaluation

We evaluate COASTmed through comparative analyses with respect to the desired properties with a representative set of technologies approaching similar challenges regarding privacy, access control, and customization. These are either healthcare specific or appropriate for the healthcare context. We assess their ability to allow a provider to (a) expressively capture privacy and operational policies, (b) offer policy compliant services; (c) provide user-specific services, and (d) allow service customization to enable users to manipulate the service to fit their needs within the granted functionality. In doing so, we gain insight on how COASTmed is superior and not just different. This evaluation is limited to functional capabilities and excludes usability and user interface aspects.

3.1 Systems Overview

Cassandra is a policy language and an authorization and trust management system for establishing trust between strangers [6]. Cassandra supports role-based access control based on subject attributes. Its policy language provides built-in syntax for role activation and deactivation, registration-authority-issued credential request, and action execution. Automated remote credential retrieval is the foundation for trust management, and therefore supported. At users' request, policies are evaluated and access control decisions are made accordingly.

Haas et al. propose a privacy aware system where patients define privacy policies to control the disclosure of their data held by EHR storage agencies [7]. Data is tied to provenance information (patient identity, data consumer and provider, and relevant policies). Patients do not need to trust data holders; data access is forbidden unless explicitly authorized. Patients can audit and trace disclosed data to detect policy violations; data providers cannot repudiate unauthorized disclosures recorded in logs and data tags. Data consumers may disclose data to other parties by tagging data with new consumers' identities. Enabling mechanisms are digital watermarks and fingerprints.

InfoShare addresses the unavailability of remotely dispersed patient history at the point of care [8]. InfoShare is an access control model and policy scheme for sharing discrete and aggregated EHR data, considering source-specific disclosure policies. Patients authorize access to their records held by diverse data providers and consumers can obtain EHRs "views" on-the-fly by aggregating authorized data. Conflicting multi-source policies are resolved in the aggregation process. Unauthorized disclosures are prevented by filtering data from records based on data properties, thus requests are only matched with authorized data.

OASIS is a RBAC access control model supporting decentralized role management, parameterized roles, and role appointment [9]. Distributed resources are exposed as OASIS services within an event-based architecture. At a service request, user credentials are checked against role membership policies, activating roles accordingly and granting access to authorized services. Parameterized roles bestow finer-grained privileges and permit defining exceptions to default role privileges. Parameters may include computer id, role activator, group membership, pre-requisite roles, and environment conditions (e.g., date). OASIS is used in a national health system where EHR fragments are retrieved from a network of decentralized healthcare providers to obtain integrated patient data. Requests are anonymous due to privacy—providers cannot know their origin.

PERMIS PMI is a policy-driven, role-based privilege management infrastructure [10]. Policies define recognized system roles, privileges assigned to roles, conditions on those privileges, and authorized parties to assign roles. Policies—stored within LDAP directories—include (a) subject domains; (b) roles; (c) trusted authorities to assign roles to subjects; (d) roles to subjects assignments; (e) target domains; (f) parameterized actions supported by targets; (g) roles, actions, and targets associations and access conditions. To access services, the PERMIS decision engine checks user roles against policies—both fetched from configured LDAP directories—to accordingly make access control decisions. PERMIS has been used for the electronic transmission of drug prescriptions.

A **Privacy and Access Control for IHE-Based Systems**, supporting healthcare domain ontologies and communication standards (e.g., IHE and HL7), is proposed by Katt et al. [11]. Both access control (maps user roles to document types) and privacy policies (patients' preferences on data disclosure) are supported. A patient's EHR is a collection of *resource objects* distributed among various *domains*. EHR, however, are perceived as a unified virtual resource. At a user's request, a *decision request* is sent to a central *Policy Decision Point (PDP)*, which fetches a patient's privacy policy. A *permit* decision is made if the user is entitled to the entire EHR and each EHR portion is fetched by each *responding domain*. Otherwise, each responding domain sends a *multi-resource* request to the PDP for an individual access decision to be made based on policies so that, accordingly, specific EHR portions are returned to the requester.

Architectural Style for Pervasive Healthcare Systems. In Pervasive Healthcare systems, a network of users, wearable health sensors, PDAs, and databases dynamically exchange information [12]. The proposed architecture focuses on run-time reconfiguration given the transience of users and devices. The architecture follows the publish/subscribe style—a distributor mediates parties interactions by distributing event notifications to subscribed parties, decoupling message senders and receivers. Rule-based graph transformation and model checking methods are used to formally model and verify structure and behavior (communication mechanisms). Rules dictate the way and the circumstances for a system's reconfiguration. A *connect* graph transformation rule, for example, creates a message channel to connect a component to a distributor.

3.2 Evaluation

Most evaluated systems have a policy-based approach to the authorized disclosure of patient data, where policies are the basis for access control decisions. Various formalisms, diverse in semantics and syntax, are used to capture privacy policies—OASIS model is based on propositional logic while InfoShare uses an XPath-like notation. They also differ in the ease and clearness to specify policies. For example, InfoShare's supports the specification of both authorization and prohibition policies, requiring policy conflict resolution, while Cassandra, PERMIS, and COASTmed reduce complexity by allowing only positive policies (i.e. everything is denied unless explicitly granted). Systems also differ on who is responsible for defining policies. For example, in Haas et al. the patient is solely responsible for defining disclosure policies and the data holder has no access to data. In contrast, in COASTmed, InfoShare, and the Privacy and Access Control for IHE-Based Systems (hereafter, Katt et al.) both the data holder (e.g., a hospital) and the patient can specify data disclosure policies.

Not every evaluated system has the ability to provide services that are explicitly tied and compliant with policies. For example, in Cassandra, policy evaluation produces either an "accept" or a "deny" access decision, but it is not made explicit how access rights are bound to capabilities (presumably, access control mechanisms bind policies and services); in Haas et al. patient policies are checked against requests to, accordingly, grant or deny access to data; in Katt et al., a central policy decision point along with enforcement components within each responding domain oversee policy compliance. However, it is not clear in these systems how policies and services are tied together. In contrast, systems such as InfoShare, OASIS, PERMIS PMI, and COASTmed make explicit the association between policies and offered services. For instance, InfoShare policies explicitly point to hierarchically structured data objects returned to users; in OASIS, service access is contingent on presenting role membership certificates issued according to policies, where services are associated to roles; in PERMIS, target applications' methods and arguments are specified within access control policies; COASTmed explicitly binds policies with system functions, generates service CURLs based on the evaluated policies, and thus policies are effectively enforced. Also, comparatively, auditing technologies such as in Haas et al. have a forensic approach to the disclosure through the identification of unauthorized disclosures, while COASTmed prevents such disclosures in the first place.

Most evaluated technologies, such as Cassandra, PERMIS PMI, and Katt et al., provide role-specific services addressing user categories. However, it may

Table 1. Evaluation summary

	expressively captures policies	policy compliant services	user-specific services	customizable service
Cassandra	✓	✓	✓	✗
Haas et al.	✓	✓	✓	✗
InfoShare	✓	✓	✓	✗
OASIS	✓	✓	✓	✗
PERMIS	✓	✓	✓	✗
Katt et al.	✓	✓	✓	✗
Rafe et al.	✗	N/K	✓	✓
COASTmed	✓	✓	✓	✓

also be desirable to treat individuals distinctively despite their roles, therefore only supporting role-based access control may be limiting. In the Pervasive Healthcare Systems Architecture (hereafter, Rafe et al.), consumers subscribe to services of interest, therefore in some sense services are audience-specific, however not specific to any particular user. A more fine-grained approach to access control considers also subject identity. InfoShare, for example, provides authorized views of patient data to both roles and principals; in OASIS all privileges are associated with both roles and principals; COASTmed not only supports role based-access control, but policies can be as low level as necessary, specifying per-organization or per-individual policies according to distinctive attributes. In COASTmed, policy specification is the liaison between user roles and services.

With the exception of COASTmed, none of the evaluated systems enable user-controlled customization—services such as in PERMIS are rather coarse-grained, one-size-fits-all. In some way, Rafe et al. offers customization by allowing users to only receive notifications from events of interest, however they are not personalized nor custom; notifications are public or private, without further granularity to subscribe to and publish events. Note that while personalization is controlled by the provider, customization gives users control to some extent. OASIS also provides limited personalization through parameterized roles. COASTmed's code mobility enables customization through the composition of expressive custom closures executed by the service to obtain the required data (Table 1).

4   Discussion

The common trait of the evaluated systems is their focus on decentralization. Although some EHR solutions exhibit centralized SCADA-like architectures, these are more appropriate when rigorous control is desired as for controlling actuators and acquiring data from distributed sensors in manufacturing plants. These networks are awash in security weaknesses, have a single point of failure, and are subject to frequent attacks [13]. Moreover, they are not meant to capture processes involving complex communities of autonomous parties. They could, however, be components within larger decentralized systems such as COASTmed, for example, for controlling medical devices through policy-based services.

These technologies exhibit, however, substantial differences in goals—Katt et al. focuses on the aggregation of distributed data, while COASTmed emphasizes on how individual providers can offer services enforcing their own policies. However, they are all concerned with the authorized and secure access to patient data. An important insight provided by the evaluation is that technologies focus on either access control (some through formal policies) or on customization, whereas none of them have the dual goal of offering a secure, yet customizable service access. COASTmed stands out by simultaneously enabling differential access to services and user-controlled customization.

A significant difference between these systems and COASTmed is that access control is a process performed at every service request. For example, in Katt et al., a single request requires complex and repetitive policy checking and multiple inter-host messages to access data within distributed providers. In COASTmed, role- and identity-related policies are checked once at the initial request for service to generate a user-specific service CURL. However, time- or date-related policies or those contingent on the attributes of the specific service request require evaluation at every request. Additionally, a provider may arbitrarily deny service to a given principal just by revoking the principal-specific CURL.

Another distinctive property of COASTmed is that trust mechanisms are decentralized. COAST relies on self-certified islands along with decentralized Web of Trust (WoT) mechanisms, while approaches such as Cassandra rely on centralized certificate authorities. Also, in COASTmed, policies are local to individual healthcare providers, while in PERMIS, for example, a centralized authority such as the National Department of Health defines policies by which local services operate. Another example is Katt et al. which relies on a centralized policy repository to make access control decisions to obtain distributed data.

The evaluated systems have, however, some advantages over COASTmed and features worth adopting in future work. For example, Cassandra considers the exchange and combination of inter-organizational policies; Haas et al.'s approach tags data with provenance information to support the continuity of policy compliance throughout the flow of patient data; InfoShare aggregates health data from different sources, combining their individual policies and resolving conflicting ones in order to comply with all providers' privacy requirements; Katt et al. has the ability to make fine-grained access control decisions based on individual EHR documents whose fragments are dispersed among autonomous providers.

A barrier for adoption of some technologies, including COASTmed, is the complexity of formalizing policies. However, the critical nature of the information justifies this difficulty. Policy languages have undeniable advantages such as unambiguously capturing domain rules and automating policy evaluation and conflict resolution. Policies are meant to be specified by expert teams of domain policy makers and developers. Appropriate graphic user interfaces and policy reuse are needed to support policy makers in their tasks and more basic patient consent forms to make policy specification feasible in day-to-day practice.

5 Conclusions

We present COASTmed, an EHR management system which exhibits novel techniques to provide differential and customizable access to EHR data services. Our techniques are grounded on the architectural principles of the COAST architectural style and on the expressiveness of the Rei policy language. These enabling technologies—which include Motile/Island, COAST's implementation infrastructure—permit healthcare providers to offer computationally-enabled user-specific services that operate according to formally specified privacy and operational policies. In COASTmed, the information provider is empowered to offer fine-grained differential access to services and users can customize services within the authority granted. Our presented approach supports the secure, privacy-aware, customizable use, and decentralized sharing of patient information. These novel secure, per-user services provide a competitive and economic opportunity for healthcare providers and other organizations managing health data.

References

1. Rindfleisch, T.C.: Privacy, information technology, and health care. Commun. ACM **40**(8), 92–100 (1997)
2. Gorlick, M.M., Strasser, K., Taylor, R.N.: Coast: an architectural style for decentralized on-demand tailored services. In: Joint Working IEEE/IFIP Conference on Software Architecture and European Conference on Software Architecture, pp. 71–80 (2012)
3. Alhaqbani, B., Fidge, C.: Access control requirements for processing electronic health records. In: Hofstede, A., Benatallah, B., Paik, H.-Y. (eds.) BPM 2007. LNCS, vol. 4928, pp. 371–382. Springer, Heidelberg (2008). doi:10.1007/978-3-540-78238-4_38
4. Gorlick, M.M., Taylor, R.N.: Communication and capability URLs in COAST-based decentralized services. In: Pautasso, C., Wilde, E., Alarcon, R. (eds.) REST: Advanced Research Topics and Practical Applications, pp. 9–25. Springer, New York (2014). doi:10.1007/978-1-4614-9299-3_2
5. Kagal, L., Finin, T., Joshi, A.: A policy based approach to security for the semantic web. In: Fensel, D., Sycara, K., Mylopoulos, J. (eds.) ISWC 2003. LNCS, vol. 2870, pp. 402–418. Springer, Heidelberg (2003). doi:10.1007/978-3-540-39718-2_26
6. Becker, M.Y., Sewell, P.: Cassandra: flexible trust management, applied to electronic health records. In: Proceedings of the 17th IEEE Computer Security Foundations Workshop, pp. 139–154 (2004)
7. Haas, S., Wohlgemuth, S., Echizen, I., Sonehara, N., Mller, G.: Aspects of privacy for electronic health records. Int. J. Med. Inform. **80**(2), e26–e31 (2011)

8. Jin, J., Covington, M.J., Ahn, G., Hu, H., Zhang, X.: Patient-centric authorization framework for sharing electronic health records. In: ACM SACMAT, pp. 125–134 (2009)

9. Eyers, D.M., Bacon, J., Moody, K.: OASIS role-based access control for electronic health records. IEE Proc. Softw. **153**(1), 16–23 (2006)

10. Chadwick, D., Mundy, D.: Policy based electronic transmission of prescriptions. In: Proceedings of the IEEE 4th International Workshop on Policies for Distributed Systems and Networks, POLICY 2003, pp. 197–206 (2003)

11. Katt, B., Breu, R., Hafner, M., Schabetsberger, T., Mair, R., Wozak, F.: Privacy and access control for IHE-based systems. In: Weerasinghe, D. (ed.) eHealth 2008. LNICSSITE, vol. 0001, pp. 145–153. Springer, Heidelberg (2009). doi:10. 1007/978-3-642-00413-1_18

12. Rafe, V., Hajvali, M.: Designing an architectural style for pervasive healthcare systems. J. Med. Syst. **37**(2), 1–13 (2013)

13. Igure, V.M., Laughter, S.A., Williams, R.D.: Security issues in SCADA networks. Comput. Secur. **25**(7), 498–506 (2006)

Process Execution and Enactment
in Medical Environments

Bernard Lambeau[✉], Christophe Damas, and Axel van Lamsweerde

ICTEAM Research Institute, Université catholique de Louvain, Louvain-la-Neuve, Belgium
{bernard.lambeau,christophe.damas,
axel.vanlamsweerde}@uclouvain.be

Abstract. Process models are increasingly recognized as an important asset for higher-quality healthcare. They may be used for analyzing, documenting, and explaining complex medical processes to the stakeholders involved in the process. Models may also be used for driving single processes or for orchestrating multiple ones. Model-driven software technologies therefore appear promising. In particular, process enactment provides software-based support for executing operational processes. A wide variety of possible enactment schemes are available in medical environments, e.g., to maintain daily medical worklists, to issue warnings or reminders in specific process states, to schedule tasks competing for resources, to provide on-the-fly advice in case of staff unavailability, and so forth. Such variety of possible process enactments calls for a common conceptual framework for defining, comparing, classifying, and integrating them. The paper introduces such a framework and describes a number of patterns for process execution and enactment based on it. These patterns result from a simple generic, goal-oriented model of medical process execution aiming at clarifying the role of software within the process and its environment. The patterns are illustrated on two real, non-trivial case studies.

1 Introduction

Process support is often advocated as a means for achieving higher-quality healthcare [8, 20]. In particular, medical *guidelines* capture evidence-based practices for handling specific diseases [13]; *clinical pathways* provide a patient-centric view of medical treatments involving multi-disciplinary teams, such as cancer treatments [28].

Models in this context enable the analysis, documentation and explanation of medical processes; they provide the basis for automated process support. Many languages and techniques are available for process modeling and analysis [17, 18], including UML activity diagrams [23], YAWL [31], BPMN [24], Little-JIL [4, 5, 34], and g-HMSC [9, 10].

Enactment techniques appear promising for process support in medical environments. Process *enactment* is commonly defined as the use of software to support the execution of operational processes [12, 25, 30]. In *model-driven* enactment, a high-level process model is used as input for execution support. An execution semantics of the modeling language must then be provided. For instance, YAWL has an execution

© Springer International Publishing AG 2017
M. Huhn and L. Williams (Eds.): FHIES 2014/SEHC 2014, LNCS 9062, pp. 145–161, 2017.
DOI: 10.1007/978-3-319-63194-3_10

semantics in terms of Petri nets [31]. The Business Process Execution Language (BPEL) similarly complements BPMN while focusing on web service invocation [1].

Various process enactment schemes are available in medical environments, e.g., to dynamically maintain medical worklists, issue warnings or reminders in specific process states, schedule tasks competing for resources, or provide on-the-fly medical advice.

Our experience in a variety of medical environments suggests that specific model-driven enactment schemes are effective in specific contexts only. For example, one scheme may appear appropriate for supporting daily operations in a radiotherapy department while less appropriate for enforcing the clinical pathway for stroke treatment. In the former case, the model may focus on daily tasks to be handled by medical staff within a single department; in the latter case, the model may focus on highly time-critical tasks to be coordinated among multiple departments.

In order to better understand the fundamental nature of medical process enactment and integrate the diversity of possible enactment schemes, the paper introduces a conceptual framework for process execution and enactment. This framework is based on a goal-oriented, multi-view model of process execution that highlights the role of specific agents, including software, in executing medical processes. The model is parameterized on tasks; it separates the operational process being executed within some environment from the software supporting such execution. More specifically, this model integrates a goal model underlying process execution, a companion structural model relating all concepts involved in the goal model, and a behavior model derived from the goal model that highlights execution states and transitions on which software enactors may be anchored.

The proposed framework may be used for defining, comparing, classifying or integrating various enactment strategies. In particular, patterns are defined in this framework as common forms of process execution and enactment. The framework is intended for process analysts and software engineers to reason about the introduction of software enactors for process support.

The paper is organized as follows. Section 2 summarizes some background material used in the next sections. Section 3 describes our multi-view model for process execution and enactment. Section 4 analyzes generic assets used in medical task performance together with common patterns of process execution and enactment; these assets and patterns are obtained by instantiating the multi-view model on specific tasks. Section 5 briefly discusses two real medical case studies we were involved in that illustrate some of these patterns.

2   Background: Modeling Medical Processes

Guarded High-level Message Sequence Charts (g-HMCS) are used in the paper for modeling medical processes. The g-HMSC language is a simple flowchart-style formalism for modeling multi-agent processes involving *decisions* on process variables [9]. An *agent* is an active system component playing a specific role in the considered process. Agents cooperate to satisfy the medical objectives assigned to them [19]; they can be humans, devices or software.

The g-HMSC language is used for formal analyses while being close to the informal sketches provided by medical stakeholders [10]. As Fig. 1 suggests, a g-HMSC model is a directed graph with three types of nodes.

- A *task node* captures a process task, that is, a work unit performed by collaboration of agent instances involved in the process. It is represented by a box. The arcs connecting task nodes specify how these nodes must be composed sequentially.
  A task may be *refined* in another g-HMSC. A non-refined task (or *leaf* task) is specified through a scenario showing the temporal sequence of interaction events among agent instances. Leaf tasks are considered here as black-box execution units under responsibility of a specific agent. The latter is called task *performer*. When multiple agents are involved in the same task, available mechanisms for refining agents, tasks, and their underlying objectives should be used for capturing multiple performers [19]; lack of space prevents us from considering this further here.
- A *decision node* captures a process decision. The latter states specific conditions on process variables [10] for tasks along outgoing branches to be performed.
- *Initial* and *terminal* nodes represent the start and end of the (sub-)process.

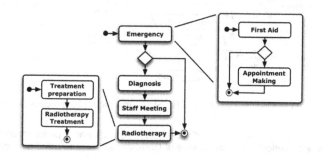

Fig. 1. A simple g-HMSC process model for cancer radiotherapy

A g-HMSC task may be annotated with additional information such as its precondition for application, its minimum/maximum duration, the resources required, and so forth [10].

3 Modeling Process Execution and Enactment

Section 3.1 introduces a generic goal model for process execution in a multi-agent setting together with a structural model interrelating the concepts involved in it. Section 3.2 discusses a corresponding behavior model highlighting execution states of process tasks together with transitions among those states. These transitions define the specific places at which software agents can be introduced for process enactment.

3.1   A Goal Model for Process Execution

This section aims at clarifying what a medical process enactor should actually be doing and why it should do so. A generic goal model is built for this; its instantiation provides the basis for defining execution strategies and enactment patterns.

A goal-oriented model integrates the intentional, structural, functional, and behavioral facets of the target system in a multi-agent setting [19]. It allows, among others, requirements on cooperating agents to be derived from high-level goals.

Figure 2(a) shows the goals (in parallelograms) underlying the execution of a medical process, how they are AND-refined into subgoals (through AND-arrows), and how they are assigned to agents (in hexagons). Figure 2(b) provides a structural model (as a UML class diagram) showing how the concepts appearing in the goal model are interrelated. Precise definitions for the goals in Fig. 2 are given in Fig. 3.

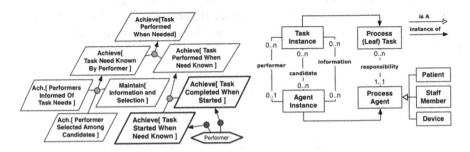

Fig. 2. (a) Generic goal model and (b) Structural model for process execution

Achieve [Task Performed When Needed]: Every task instance whose performance is needed shall eventually be performed by an instance of the responsible agent, called performer, under specific timing and resource constraints.

Achieve [Task Need Known By Performer]: For every task instance whose performance is needed, the performer shall eventually know this task instance is needed.

Achieve [Performers Informed Of Task Needs]: Every need for task performance shall eventually be known by at least one candidate performer.

Achieve [Performer Selected When Task Need]: For every task instance whose performance is needed, the actual performer shall eventually be selected among possible candidates.

Maintain Information and Selection]: Once selected a performer shall remain selected until the task is performed. Once informed a performer shall remain informed of the task performance need until the task is performed.

Achieve [Task Started When Need Known]: When the performer knows the need for performing a task instance, it shall eventually start that task so as to meet the corresponding timing and resource constraints.

Achieve [Task Completed When Started]: Every task instance whose performance has been started shall eventually be completed successfully.

Fig. 3. Specifications for the goals in Fig. 2(a)

The root goal of process enactment states that "*all task instances must eventually be performed*". (As we capture process executions, we are mostly concerned with task instances; "task performance" is often used as a shortcut for "task instance performance". Figure 2 shows a refinement-by-milestones [19] of this root goal:

- a first subgoal requires the need for performing a specific task to be known by its performer;
- once the need is known, the task shall eventually be performed.

The first subgoal is further refined. A *divide-and-conquer* refinement [19] is used:

- potential task performers shall be informed of the task performance need;
- one of these shall be selected as performer;
- agent selection and information shall not be undone.

The latter subgoal is set as an assumption to simplify matters. "Informed" and "selected" mean that if a task is performed then its performer knew that it was needed and that it was the one responsible for the task, respectively. The divide-and-conquer strategy is taken to cover various process execution scenarios, e.g. "selecting then informing" or "making all candidates informed and then selecting among them". In any case, a state must eventually be reached where the performer is both selected and informed.

The second subgoal of the root goal in Fig. 2 is refined as follows:

- the task performance shall first be started;
- it shall eventually be completed when started.

The goal model in Fig. 2 calls for further clarifications.

- The tasks to be performed there correspond to instances of *leaf* tasks in the process model; the structuring of the process model through task refinements has no impact on process executions.
- The goals of the generic model for process execution in Fig. 2 should not be confused with the objectives underlying process tasks. For example, the process model in Fig. 1 has underlying objectives such as **Achieve** [Treatment Prepared When Patient Registered] or **Maintain** [Patient Registered Before Radiotherapy]. The latter objectives are structured and refined in a specific goal model complementing the g-HMSC task model. Synergetic links exist between the treatment-specific and generic goal models; there are however not the primary focus of this paper.
- As specified in Fig. 2, the goal of a task being actually performed is assigned to the task performer. This requires the medical objective underlying the task to be *realizable* by the agent, that is, the agent must have the capabilities of *monitoring* the conditions to be evaluated and of *controlling* the conditions to be established according to this objective [19]. Agents playing the *Performer* role might be the target patient, members of the medical staff (e.g., nurse, oncologist), medical devices (e.g., pump, radiotherapy machine) or available software (e.g., patient record system).
- The three other leaf goals in Fig. 2 should be further refined to specify how task performers and software enactors cooperate in order to satisfy them. Various alternative refinements lead to various enactment patterns, see Sect. 4.

- The model is deliberately kept simple for the purpose of this paper. It can easily be extended for capturing multiple task performers, through the agent/goal refinement mechanism [19], and exceptions, through obstacle analysis [19].

3.2   A Behavior Model for Process Execution

The various execution milestones identified in our generic goal model lead to the behavior model captured as a UML state diagram in Fig. 4. Three main execution states are identified.

- *Created*: Every task instance enters this state as soon as a new process instance is started. As a process may involve multiple decisions, some task instances might not be performed in practice even though they conceptually exist.
- *PerformanceNeeded*: Every task instance is in this state when its performance need is confirmed (in a way to be made further precise). This state is further decomposed in a way consistent with the goal model.
- *Performed:* Every task instance whose performance has been completed by its performer ends up in this state.

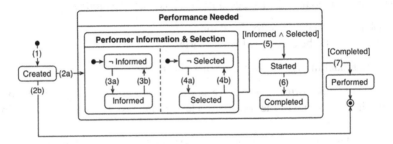

Fig. 4. States and transitions in the execution of a task instance

This behavior model is generic on tasks to be performed. Its transitions are therefore not labeled with events and/or actions; they are simply identified by a number. The guards there are derived from the goal model [19]; additional guards may be introduced when instantiating the model.

The state transitions in this behavior model yield the various places where software enactor agents may be introduced to drive the medical process. These transitions are discussed successively, focusing on *when* the transition gets fired and *how* enactment software may be involved. This paves the way to enactment patterns in Sect. 4.

(1)   *A task instance gets created as soon as a process instance is started.* Model-driven enactors typically use the process model to create task instances for further driving, thereby firing this transition.

(2a) *The need for task performance gets confirmed; the information and selection subprocesses of a task performer start accordingly.* This transition gets fired as soon as a process agent knows that performing a medical task is needed. The agent might be the patient deciding to go for consultation, the doctor prescribing some medical test, etc. In such cases, software enactors mostly help tracking corresponding needs. They might also help firing this transition by introducing effective *need identification means*.

(2b) *Task performance is not required; execution ends up immediately.* This transition accounts for task instances that conceptually exist but are not executed due to process decisions.

(3a) *The performer gets informed of the need to perform the task.* Various situations may correspond to this transition getting fired. The performer might be the one who identified the need –in which case he/she/it gets automatically informed. Alternatively, the agent might be informed by a specific request –such as a phone call, for example. Software enactors might help firing this transition by introducing effective *information means*.

(3b) *The performer gets unaware of the need to perform the task.* This transition is introduced to account for exceptional situations where, e.g., performers forget about their task commitments. Software enactors might help avoid this transition from getting fired by introducing effective *remembering means*.

(4a) *The performer gets selected among possible candidates.* This transition is fired as soon as the agent instance to actually perform the task is known. In simple situations with only one candidate or a predetermined selection result, the transition gets fired automatically without requiring any kind of support. Otherwise, software enactors might help firing this transition by introducing effective *selection means*.

(4b) *The selected performer gets unselected.* This transition is introduced to account for exceptional situations where, e.g., selected performers suddenly get unavailable –introducing the risk of tasks being not performed or performed too late. Enactors might be introduced to detect such situations and mitigate their consequences.

(5) *The task performance gets started under the necessary condition that the performer is both selected and informed.* In our framework, the responsibility of starting a task is assigned to its performer. A *trigger condition* should capture when the transition gets fired, e.g., "as soon as the performer is available" or "at some predefined moment". Software enactors may help performers here.

- As seen before, effective *remembering* and *selection means* help keeping the guard satisfied for tasks whose performance is needed.
- *Prioritizing means* may help selecting which task instances to perform among those having their transition currently enabled.

(6) *The performer completes task performance.* Here again, the responsibility for task completion is assigned to the performer. Software enactors may assist here in achieving the task's post-condition (e.g., automated checklists) or in detecting task instances whose performance has started but has not been completed yet.

(7) *As the task has been completed its performance is no longer needed.* This transition captures that the performing agent gets informed that the completed task is no longer needed. In many cases, this transition is automatic; it results from the performing agent being aware of task completion. When software enactors are involved, the transition is required for enactors to be informed of tasks being no

longer needed, e.g., to remove them from task lists or to determine subsequent tasks to be performed. This may prove challenging as a feedback loop is required from performers to enactors [3, 7]. An explicit feedback requires performers to inform enactors; an implicit one uses some *monitoring means*.

4   Patterns of Process Execution and Enactment

The intentional, structural and behavior models of process execution in Sect. 3 allow us to identify patterns commonly found for getting tasks performed under specific timing and resource constraints. When software enactors are introduced, such patterns may be called *enactment* patterns. An execution/enactment pattern relies on specific task performance *assets*. Section 4.1 reviews such assets by instantiation of the concepts introduced in Sect. 3.2 –such as *information means*, *remembering means* or *trigger condition*. Assets are not necessarily independent from each other; patterns for using them together may therefore be identified. Section 4.2 lists various examples of how assets may be combined in such patterns.

4.1   Task Performance Assets

The firing means for the successive state transitions in Sect. 3.2 are instantiated with a particular focus on software enactors. The process in Fig. 1 is used as a running example for illustrating various cases.

Need identification means: How is a task known to be needed?
Symptoms or accidents may cause patients to enter a medical process. In Fig. 1, the Surgery task might be needed because of a patient feeling some specific pain. The need for performing a task may also result from a medical decision or a diagnosis made by some medical actor. For example, after the First Aid task in Fig. 1, cancer suspicion may raise the need for further diagnosis with appointments being made accordingly.

Software-aided diagnosis therefore falls into this category of process enactment [16]. *Patient monitoring systems* inside or outside the hospital might be seen as enactors too for the same reason [3, 15, 32].

Another source for identifying task needs is provided by medical guidelines. *Rule-based* or *procedural process models* formalizing guidelines may be used as assets for driving processes through dedicated enactors [22]. In such cases, the execution semantics of the modeling formalism prescribes how the software can infer which task is needed in the current process state.

Information means: How does the performer know that the task is needed?
Various information means are available for informing potential performers of tasks to be performed.

– Direct or indirect *requests* (e.g. phone calls, messages) are a usual way of informing performers of tasks to be done. For example, the Appointment Making task in Fig. 1 might simply consist in asking someone at the department's welcome desk.

- *Calendars* are another means for keeping track of tasks to be performed. For cancer treatment, for example, nurses or assistants may fill in the radiotherapist's e-calendar with specific dates for the Diagnosis task (see Fig. 1). The patient may also keep track of the dates of her Radiotherapy treatments in her own calendar.
- *Registration lists* are sometimes used for recurrent task instances. A registration list might be filled in by nurses or assistants to inform radiotherapists and oncologists of the patients to be discussed at the next multidisciplinary Staff Meeting task instance (see Fig. 1).
- *Worklists* may also be used for keeping track of tasks to be performed and informing agents about these. They might be physical ones or managed by software. For example, the medical staff might know that a new Emergency task instance in Fig. 1 is needed by looking at the physical waiting queue. The Treatment Preparation task might rely on a digital worklist for organizing the preparation of preplanned radiotherapy treatments.

Automated worklists are frequently mentioned in the literature; they originate from agenda management systems [14, 21]. Most workflow management systems actually depend on such lists for enacting process models, see e.g. [2, 33, 34].

Remembering means: *How does the performer remember that the task is needed?*
Most information means may also be used as remembering means –in particular, calendars, registration lists and worklists.

- *Reminders* are also commonly used in medical practice [16]. They can be easily automated for tasks whose performance time is known in advance –e.g., from the Diagnosis appointment known from the medical e-agenda (see Fig. 1). When effective *identification* and *information means* are available, more complex reminding schemes can be implemented. For example, a reminder to participate to the next Staff Meeting task might be automatically sent to the Radiologist only under the condition that at least one of her patients appears on the registration list.

Selection means: *How is the performer selected among candidates for the task?*
In situations where the assignment of tasks to performer instances is not necessarily obvious, various selection strategies are available.

- The *first-available-performer* strategy accounts for situations where a pool of performer instances process tasks as the flow is going. This strategy is commonly used when a worklist is used as information means –e.g. as in the Emergency task, or in the Treatment Preparation task that might involve a pool of physicists acting according to a digital worklist (see Sect. 5.1).
- *Static allocation* assigns tasks to performers on a pre-established basis. For example, chemotherapy treatments might be organized according to a pre-established assignment of beds to nurses.
- *Dynamic allocation* assigns tasks according to resource availability and other constraints. Performer instances do not decide which task instances they perform. Software may be used here for enactment and sometimes for task performance. The

automated scheduling of Radiotherapy Treatments according to available treatment machines is an example of this.

Selection means are not intended to make dynamic choices among agent instances based on their respective role or capabilities; this is achieved at modeling time through the introduction of different agents with specific roles, capabilities, and responsibility assignments [19].

Prioritizing means: *How are task instances selected for performance?*
While *selection means* prescribe how performers are selected, *prioritizing means* prescribe in what order the latter perform tasks among those needed. Prioritizing means are commonly used when task instances compete for resource availability.

- *First-In-First-Out*: This static strategy is often used in combination with pure queue-based worklists –see, e.g., the Appointment Making task in Fig. 1. Registration lists sometimes implement this strategy as well.
- *Highest-Priority-First:* This dynamic strategy is also frequently used in combination with worklists and registration lists –e.g., to account for urgency in the Emergency task or in Staff Meeting discussions. Software enactors might be introduced here as well. For example, instances of the Treatment Preparation task in Fig. 1 might be dynamically prioritized in a worklist according to known dates for the corresponding Radiotherapy Treatment.
- *Automated Scheduling:* Prioritization with dynamic performer allocation under complex constraints may require an *online* or an *offline* scheduler. This software enactor computes what tasks are to be performed first, either on the fly (online) or ahead of time (offline).

Trigger conditions: *What makes tasks getting started?*
In correlation with the *information*, *remembering*, *selection* and/or *prioritizing* means, task instances occur at a specific time and/or for specific reasons. Provided the required resources are available and the task's precondition is met, the following conditions may trigger task performance.

- *As-Soon-As*: When a request or a worklist is used as information means, tasks are sometimes performed as soon as the selected performer instance is available. This might for example be the case for the Appointment Making task in Fig. 1.
- *Highest-Priority*: When prioritization means are used, a task may start as soon as it gets the highest priority. The First Aid and Treatment Preparation tasks in Fig. 1 are typical examples of this.
- *Fixed-Time*: Many medical tasks simply occur at some fixed, predetermined time. In Fig. 1, the Diagnosis task might occur according to a predetermined appointment. Radiotherapy Treatments similarly follow a pre-established schedule. Staff Meeting instances generally occur at a specific time slot every week.

4.2   Combining Performance Assets: Process Execution/Enactment Patterns

Figure 5 shows a number of typical patterns obtained when performance assets are combined. Those patterns provide a way of explaining why tasks are actually performed in practice and how software enactors may support process execution. The list of identified patterns is obviously not exhaustive.

		Request-driven	Appointment-driven	Meeting-driven	Priority-driven	Resource-driven	Scheduling-driven
Information	Request	x					
	Calendar		x				
	Registration list			x			
	Worklist				x	x	
Selection	First available						
	Static allocation		x				
	Dynamic allocation						x
Prioritizing	FIFO	x					
	Priorities				x		
	Scheduling						x
Trigger	As soon as	x				x	
	Highest priority				x		
	Fixed time		x	x			

Fig. 5. Combining assets: process execution and enactment patterns

Request-driven: This pattern refers to situations where a task is performed on request, as soon as its performer is available, and in a first-in-first-out order. It might capture how tasks are performed at a welcome desk or how requests issued by bedridden patients are handled. The Appointment Making task in Fig. 1 follows this pattern.

Appointment-driven: This pattern refers to tasks such as Diagnosis or Consultation. For such tasks, calendars are used by performers to agree and remember fixed-time appointments. Most often, the performer is statically known as in the case of Consultation with a specialist. Support for e-calendars accessible to medical staff is then an effective form of enactment.

Meeting-driven: This pattern refers to tasks such as Staff (see Fig. 1) or Support Group Meetings. Such meetings occur at a fixed, recurrent time –e.g., once a week. Registration lists are used to track which patients must be discussed or need be present. Automating such lists and the registration process results in effective information and remembering means.

Priority-driven: Automated worklists correspond to a well-known kind of model-driven process enactment. An associated pattern uses priorities to decide which task instances must be performed first among those in the worklist. This pattern is compatible with all assets for performer selection. However, it assumes that performers are immediately available after having performed a task. The pattern is therefore better suited for automated performers such as medical devices. Hospital pharmacy automation provides a good example of use.

Resource-driven: This pattern is a variant of the previous one. It also relies on worklists as information means. Task performance is not driven by priorities here but by the availability of scarce resources such as the performer itself; the tasks are performed as soon as the required resources get available. The pattern is compatible with various

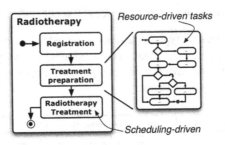

Fig. 6. Simplified radiotherapy process

prioritizing and *selection* means. The Treatment Preparation task in Fig. 1 is an example of application (see also Sect. 5.1).

Scheduling-driven: This pattern is frequently used when multiple instances of a task compete for scarce and/or costly resources. The dynamic allocation of those resources using available scheduling techniques is an effective enactment strategy in such cases. The scheduling of sessions on radiotherapy machines typically relies on this pattern (see Sect. 5.1). The determination of patient appointments under complex resource and time constraints may also benefit from this pattern (see Sect. 5.2). The scheduling may involve real-time slots decided ahead of task performance. In such cases, the pattern also relies on calendars and fixed-time appointments.

5   Case Studies

This section briefly reports on two quite different instantiations of the multi-view model in Sect. 3 and patterns in Sect. 4. These instantiations capture the effective enactment of complex processes in real medical environments. Section 5.1 refers to a software-managed daily worklist for the preparation of radiotherapy treatments. Section 5.2 outlines a tool for automated scheduling of appointments for chemotherapy treatments. Both examples are taken from real medical projects we were involved in at the UCL university hospital in Brussels.

5.1   Automated Worklist for Preparing Radiotherapy Treatments

Figure 6 shows a simplified process model for the preparation of radiotherapy treatments. A patient enters the process once her cancer has been confirmed by earlier diagnosis. The process starts with an administrative Registration task. In particular, the dates of the treatment on a specific therapy machine are scheduled at registration time. The reason is that radiotherapy machines are heavily contentious resources. A *scheduling-driven* enactment pattern is therefore used for determining the treatment dates and machines allocated for the Radiotherapy Treatment task.

This yields a specific problem for the Treatment Preparation task. For a given patient, radiotherapy preparation has a strict deadline of *14* days due to specific constraints not discussed here. The Treatment Preparation task is decomposed into subtasks handled by medical staff. (These subtasks are not detailed here for lack of space.) None of these subtasks requires the patient to be present; some require a physicist, others an assistant, and others a radiotherapist. For a given set of patients to be treated, with corresponding process instances, a daily problem is to avoid rescheduling radiotherapy sessions dynamically (to save costs). The preparation must therefore be organized so as to meet all deadlines and constraints.

An effective enactment solution consists of using an automated worklist for the Treatment Preparation subtasks, according to the *resource-driven* pattern. A software enactor implementing this pattern is used daily at the radiotherapy department of the UCL university hospital.

- The *information means* are given by the automated worklist itself. All tasks to be performed are known by the multi-disciplinary team. The worklist is however filtered by medical role.
- Various *selection means* are possible with this pattern. Here, *static allocation* on a per-patient basis is used for tasks handled by medical assistants. In contrast, physicists are selected according to the *first-available-performer* strategy.
- The actual performance of tasks is driven by resource availability. In the ideal case, a subtask is performed as soon as a performer is available (*trigger condition*) provided the task gets the highest priority (*prioritizing*). Priorities are carefully determined according to: (a) the deadline imposed by scheduling on treatment machines, and (b) statistics about the time taken by each subtask.
- To push the currently implemented approach further, a prototype tool was developed for *model-driven* enactment. A g-HMSC model of the Treatment Preparation subprocess was used to fill in and dynamically maintain the worklist automatically (*identification means*).

In terms of the state diagram in Fig. 5, transitions (2a), (2b) and (7) require some dedicated treatment through collaboration between medical staff and the software enactor. Transition (7) requires medical staff to explicit mark tasks as done in the worklist. This allows the enactor to remove these and replace them by successor tasks according to the process model –thereby firing transitions (2a) and (2b).

5.2 Scheduling Chemotherapy Treatments

A process model for simple chemotherapy-based cancer treatment is sketched in Fig. 7. While apparently similar to the previous one, the enactment solution we are developing is fairly different here.

Cancer is treated through a series of several sessions (or *cycles*) of chemotherapy treatment over a few months. Various treatment plans are available according to the kind of cancer, the patient's age, the drugs to be used, and so forth. For instance, a FEC chemotherapy cycle for treating breast cancer takes about 21 days [26]. On the first day of each cycle, the patient goes to hospital for an injection of FEC chemotherapy drugs (Delivery task in Fig. 7). Then, she has no chemotherapy for the next 20 days (Rest Period in Fig. 7). Four to six similar cycles are followed. Depending on the treatment plan, the Delivery task takes from a few minutes to a few hours. Subtasks include a

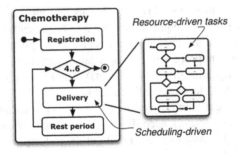

Fig. 7. Simplified chemotherapy process

consultation with an oncology assistant, drug preparation by the hospital's pharmacy, and drug injection by a nurse in some bed (to be determined). These Delivery subtasks are all driven by resource availability.

Unlike the previous case study, the problem here is not to help with the organization of those subtasks *per se*. Instead, the date of each Delivery task instance should be determined for the entire patient population –taking into account that different patients follow different treatment plans requiring different resources such as nurses, assistants, or beds; the latter are available in limited number.

The date of the first treatment is determined during the Registration task. Dates for the next treatments are determined at the end of each Delivery task. Some flexibility is provided to the patient for picking up those dates. For the treatment to be successful, however, the length of each cycle must be kept as close as possible to the one prescribed in the treatment plan.

A software enactment solution is currently being developed in our research group in collaboration with a medical team at the day care department of the UCL university hospital. It consists in scheduling drug Delivery task instances among patients over time so as to meet various types of constraints (detailed hereafter).

- An electronic calendar is used as *information means*. It lets both medical staff and patients know when each Delivery instance takes place.
- *Prioritizing* is achieved using constraint-based local search technology [11]. Our scheduler generates Delivery dates for each patient so as to meet the following:
  - the corresponding process model, in particular, the time bounds on the various treatment cycles;
  - resource availability constraints;
  - a target criterion on a safety-critical process quality indicator. More specifically, the *Relative Dose Intensity* (RDI) indicator captures how close the dose actually delivered to a patient over time is to the optimal dose intensity. Roughly, the higher the RDI the closer the actual treatment is to the optimal treatment plan prescribed by the evidence-based process model.

The scheduler continuously computes "best" date proposals and fills in the e-calendar. The proposal for the next delivery date is accepted or adapted by the patient at the end of each Delivery task instance, in agreement with the medical assistant and nurse. When the proposed dates are changed in the calendar, the impact of the change on the resulting RDI is shown as feedback to patients, assistants and nurses to possibly warn them about the consequences of the change on the treatment effectiveness.

6   Conclusion

The paper presented a goal-oriented multi-view model for reasoning about medical process execution and enactment. Task performance assets and process execution/enactment patterns were identified by instantiation of this generic model. The objective was by no means to define yet another process modeling or execution language. Rather, the proposed framework provides abstract support for process analysts and software engineers to reason about medical process executions and anchor software enactors on the process. Even though the g-HMSC process modeling language is incidentally used, our conceptual framework does not really depend on a particular modeling language. Similarly, it does not presuppose any particular execution semantics.

The richness, variety and complexity of medical environments provide evidence that human-intensive processes are first and foremost executed on the field [7]. For software enactors to be effective, a fine understanding of the process environment appears a prerequisite. Experience with execution/enactment patterns suggests that they are worth reusing. Further understanding of the nature of medical process execution should yield more patterns and increase their effectiveness.

As mentioned before, the simple conceptual framework in this paper may easily be extended to capture multiple agents cooperating to the same task; the available mechanisms for refining goals, agent, assignments and tasks may be used for this [9, 10, 19]. Resources and their capabilities should also be brought explicitly into the framework [27]. Exceptions need to be more thoroughly considered [29]; currently, only cases of tasks being forgotten or performers being unavailable are covered. Systematic obstacle analysis [19] against leaf goals in our multi-view execution model would integrate exceptional situations where tasks are cancelled, resources are unavailable, task pre- or postconditions are violated, and so forth. This would result in a more comprehensive and robust behavioral model with new corresponding states and transitions. New software enactors could then be plugged in for those transitions, and new patterns identified accordingly. For instance, anchoring the detection of deviations from the normal process [6] would require transitions capturing tasks being forgotten or cancelled.

Process modeling requires the underlying process goals, expectations on human agents, and requirements on medical devices to be structured in a process-specific goal model. The execution/enactment patterns in practice depend on such goals and their potential obstacles. Future work should therefore be devoted to the synergetic links between the process model and its companion goal model on the one hand, and their relation to the generic execution framework and enactment patterns outlined here on the other hand.

Acknowledgement. We wish to thank P. Scalliet and M. Coevoet for providing us with details about their radiotherapy worklist software outlined in Sect. 5.1. Many thanks are also due to R.

De Landtsheer, F. Roucoux, Y. Guyot, C. Ponsard and Y. Humblet for their collaboration in designing the scheduling engine in Sect. 5.2. This work was supported by the Regional Government of Wallonia (PIPAS project Nr. 1017087).

References

1. Andrews, T., et al.: Business Process Execution Language for Web Services, Version 1.1, May 2003. See also OASIS Standard WS-BPEL 2.0

2. Anzböck, R., Dustdar, S.: Modeling and implementing medical web services. Data Knowl. Eng. **55**(2), 203–236 (2005)

3. Behnam, S.A., Badreddin, O.: Toward a care process metamodel for business intelligence healthcare monitoring solutions. In: Proceedings of 5th International Workshop on Software Engineering in Health Care (SEHC 2013), pp. 79–85 (2013)

4. Chen, B., Avrunin, G.S., Henneman, E.A., Clarke, L.A., Osterweil, L.J., Henneman, P.L.: Analyzing medical processes. In: Proceedings of the 30th International Conference on Software Engineering (ICSE 2008). ACM-IEEE, pp. 623–632 (2008)

5. Christov, S., et al.: Rigorously defining and analyzing medical processes: an experience report. In: Giese, H. (ed.) MODELS 2007. LNCS, vol. 5002, pp. 118–131. Springer, Heidelberg (2008). doi:10.1007/978-3-540-69073-3_14

6. Christov, S.C., Avrunin, G.S., Clarke, L.A.: Considerations for online deviation detection in medical processes. In: Proceedings of the 5th International Workshop on Software Engineering in Health Care (SEHC 2013), pp. 50–56 (2013)

7. Clarke, L.A., Osterweil, L.J., Avrunin, G.S.: Supporting human-intensive systems. In: Proceedings of FSE/SDP Workshop on Future of Software Engineering Research, pp. 87–92 (2010)

8. Dadam, P., Reichert, M., Kuhn, K.: Clinical Workflows—The Killer Application for Process-Oriented Information Systems? pp. 36–59. Springer, London (2000)

9. Damas, C., Lambeau, B., Roucoux, F., van Lamsweerde, A.: Analyzing critical process models through behavior model synthesis. In: Proceedings of the 31st International Conference on Software Engineering (ICSE 2009), Vancouver, pp. 441–451 (2009)

10. Damas, C., Lambeau, B., van Lamsweerde, A.: Analyzing critical decision-based processes. IEEE Trans. Softw. Eng. **40**(4), 338–365 (2014)

11. De Landtsheer, R., Ponsard, C.: Oscar.cbls: an open source framework for constraint-based local search. In: 27th ORBEL Annual Meeting, Kortrijk, 7–8 February 2013

12. Finkelstein, A., Kramer, J., Nuseibeh, B. (eds.): Software Process Modelling and Technology. Research Studies Press Ltd., Taunton (1994)

13. Gordon, C., Veloso, M., The PRESTIGE Consortium: Guidelines in healthcare: the experience of the PRESTIGE Project, Medical Informatics Europe. IOS Press (1999)

14. Heisel, M.: Agendas – a concept to guide software development activities. In: Proceedings of the IFIP TC2 WG2: 4th Working Conference on Systems Implementation, Languages, Methods and Tools, pp. 19–32. Chapman & Hall (1998)

15. Hou, J.C.: Pas: a wireless-enabled, sensor-integrated personal assistance system for independent and assisted living. In: High Confidence Medical Devices, Software, and Systems and Medical Device Plug-and-Play Interoperability (2007)

16. Johnston, M.E., Langton, K.B., Haynes, R.B., Mathieu, A.: Effects of computer-based clinical decision support systems on clinician performance and patient outcome: a critical appraisal of research. Ann. Intern. Med. **120**(2), 135–142 (1994)

17. Jun, G.T., Ward, J.R., Morris, Z.: Health care process modelling: which method when? Int. J. Qual. Health Care **21**(3), 214–224 (2009)
18. Kaiser, S., Miksch, S.: Modeling computer-supported clinical guidelines and protocols: a survey. Vienna Univ. Technology, report Asgaard-TR-2005-2 (2005)
19. van Lamsweerde, A.: Requirements Engineering: From System Goals to UML Models to Software Specifications. Wiley, Chichester (2009)
20. Lenz, R., Reichert, M.: IT support for healthcare processes. In: Aalst, W.M.P., Benatallah, B., Casati, F., Curbera, F. (eds.) BPM 2005. LNCS, vol. 3649, pp. 354–363. Springer, Heidelberg (2005). doi:10.1007/11538394_24
21. McCall, E.K., Clarke, L.A., Osterweil, L.J.: An adaptable generation approach to agenda management. In: Proceedings of the 20th International Conference on Software Engineering (ICSE 1998), pp. 282–291 (2008)
22. Mathe, J., Sztipanovits, J., Levy, M., Jackson, E.K., Schulte, W.: Cancer treatment planning: formal methods to the rescue. In: Proceedings of the 4th International Workshop on Software Engineering in Health Care (SEHC 2012), Zurich (2012)
23. OMG: UML 2.0 Superstructure Specification (2003)
24. OMG: Business Process Modeling Notation, v1.1 (2008)
25. Osterweil, L.J.: Software processes are software too. In: Proceedings of the 9th International Conference on Software Engineering (ICSE 1987), pp. 2–13. ACM-IEEE (1987)
26. Perry, M.C.: The Chemotherapy Source Book. Lippincott Williams & Wilkins, Philadelphia (2008)
27. Raunak, M.S., Osterweil, L.J.: Resource management for complex, dynamic environments. IEEE Trans. Softw. Eng. **39**(3), 384–402 (2013)
28. Renholm, M., Leino-Kilpi, H., Suominen, T.: Critical pathways: a systematic review. J. Nurs. Adm. **32**(4), 196–202 (2002)
29. Staudt Lerner, B., Christov, S., Osterweil, L.J., Bendraou, R., Kannengiesser, U., Wise, A.: Exception handling patterns for process modeling. IEEE Trans. Softw. Eng. **36**(2), 162–183 (2010)
30. Aalst, W.M.P., Hofstede, A.H.M., Weske, M.: Business process management: a survey. In: Aalst, W.M.P., Weske, M. (eds.) BPM 2003. LNCS, vol. 2678, pp. 1–12. Springer, Heidelberg (2003). doi:10.1007/3-540-44895-0_1
31. van der Aalst, W., et al.: YAWL: yet another workflow language. Inf. Syst. **30**(4), 245–275 (2005)
32. Wang, Q., Shin, W., Liu, X., Zeng, Z., Oh, C., AlShebli, B.K.: I-living: an open system architecture for assisted living. In: SMC, pp. 4268–4275 (2006)
33. Westergaard, M., Maggi, F.M.: Declare: a tool suite for declarative workflow modeling and enactment. In: BPM (Demos), p. 820 (2011)
34. Wise, A., Cass, A.G., Lerner, B.S., McCall, E.K., Osterweil, L.J., Sutton, S.M.: Using little-JIL to coordinate agents in software engineering. In: Proceedings of the Automated Software Engineering Conference (ASE 2000), Grenoble, pp. 155–163. IEEE (2000)

Engineering a Performance Management System to Support Community Care Delivery

Pillar Mata[1], Craig Kuziemsky[1(✉)], Jaspreet Singh[1],
Aladdin Baarah[2], and Liam Peyton[1]

[1] University of Ottawa, Ottawa, Canada
pilimata@hotmail.com, kuziemsky@telfer.uottawa.ca,
{jbind059,lpeyton}@uottawa.ca
[2] Hashemite University, Zarqa, Jordan
aladdin.baarah@hu.edu.jo

Abstract. The engineering of health information technology (HIT) often focuses on clinical or hospital focused tasks. As more care is provided in the community there is an increasing need to monitor goals of care related to patient care delivery. These goals are often measured through performance metrics. Before we can track performance metrics we need to articulate the data and processes that define the metrics. However, the data sources are often varied and the processes ill-defined making it hard to engineer systems to collect and analyze metrics. Further, the ability to share data between organizations is impacted by culture, technology and privacy issues. To date there are few methodological approaches for modeling a health system from the perspective of metrics, data sources, and touch points to enable performance management of community based healthcare delivery. This paper addresses those shortcomings and presents a methodology for modeling goals, metrics and data to enable engineering of business intelligence applications for performance management of community based care.

Keywords: Community based care delivery · Performance management · Business intelligence · Metrics · Processes · Monitoring · Methodology

1 Introduction

An Institute of Medicine report published in 2012 concluded that the present healthcare trajectory has become too complex and costly and that digital technology will be a key aspect of healthcare delivery [1]. Health information technology (HIT) has been advocated as a solution to assist health care authorities better provide service delivery in the context of shrinking workforces and increased need for services [2, 3]. However, to date the design of HIT has met with mixed results [4], often due to differences between the design and engineering of systems and how tasks are actually done in healthcare settings [5].

While we have made progress at engineering HIT to support clinical tasks, HIT design to support post-acute or community based care delivery remains a challenge [6]. As chronic disease becomes more prevalent it is necessary to develop HIT to support

M. Huhn and L. Williams (Eds.): FHIES 2014/SEHC 2014, LNCS 9062, pp. 162–177, 2017.
DOI: 10.1007/978-3-319-63194-3_11

continuity of care across different providers and settings [7–9]. Although a patient's care may originate and be coordinated through a hospital, many of the services a patient receives may be in the community. Poor integration of services is a huge barrier to continuity of care and can result in unintended consequences including financial, human resource, and patient safety [10, 11].

Community based HIT design introduces new challenges including disparate data sources, processes as well as system interoperability issues. The focus of systems engineering is also different in that accountability, care coordination and performance management to support health services accreditation are key objectives. As the costs of healthcare delivery have increased there is a need to monitor care delivery to ensure that resources are coordinated and deployed as efficiently as possible while also ensuring high quality patient care [12, 13]. Health services accreditation is viewed as a way to improve the quality of health care and health care delivery and the need for effective governance with respect to quality standards has been well documented [14].

The notion of performance management driven healthcare delivery is not new as detailed frameworks for the design and implementation of performance management to support hospital based care have existed for some time. These frameworks have suggested that a trajectory for performance management of healthcare activities should document processes, reduce variation and monitor performance over time [28]. However, to date these frameworks have been largely designed to support hospital based performance management. While we have made progress at designing HIT to support 'internal teams' (i.e. teams within a single boundary of patient care such a hospital) we have not made as much progress at engineering HIT to support teamwork in the community – i.e. 'external teams' [13]. Moving performance management outside traditional hospital boundaries presents additional challenges. One such challenge is because national and local strategies are often at odds with each other and HIT that have been designed to support local care delivery often do not scale up to regional or national data requirements [15, 29]. A second challenge is because of what we call the *process-data chasm*. Standards committees and governing bodies may define metrics they wish to collect to assess quality of care delivery but it can be a challenge to collect the data to instantiate the metrics because the processes that define these metrics are poorly defined, or the data itself is of poor quality, both of which makes the metrics less meaningful for providing evidence on quality of care delivery [16].

Palliative care is care of patients with a terminal illness and is provided over a continuum of care from weeks to months [17]. In the context of palliative care delivery, it is necessary to track patients across multiple settings as a patient's clinical status may impact decisions that are made in the community. For example, common goals of palliative care programs are to keep patients out of the emergency room (ER) and to not use invasive therapies like chemotherapy in the last few weeks of life [18]. There is also a desire to measure competency metrics to ensure that providers have appropriate training to provide care [19]. However, a disconnect exists between the metrics and the engineering and implementation of performance management systems in the community to collect data to measure the metrics.

To date there are few papers that have looked at how to model and engineer systems to support system level interoperability and accountability. This paper addresses that shortcoming and provides a methodology for modeling goals, metrics and data to enable engineering of business intelligence applications for performance management of community based care. We use a case example of community based palliative care delivery to provide proof of concept of our approach.

2 Background

Since 2010 we have been involved in the design of a palliative care information system called *PAL-IS*. In our initial design for PAL-IS we designed a system to support a caregiving team. The initial goals of PAL-IS were to support collaborative care delivery, patient care and service delivery [20]. From 2010–2012 we developed several prototypes of PAL-IS to achieve the desired objectives [21]. However, while we were obtaining system requirements for PAL-IS we realized that some of the requirements were not related to internal team support for palliative care delivery but rather were performance management metrics. For example, a physician in an administrator role, wanted to be able to track whether a resident was present during a consult. A nursing administrator wanted to be able to track palliative care education that was provided in the community. As we considered these change requests we realized that we needed to move from engineering a system for a *team* to engineering a system for a *region*. Further, these performance management requests were a challenge as they were not readily available from existing data. While we could add the data fields into the clinical version of PAL-IS to enter them after the fact that is not the best solution as it adds design overhead and also prevents real-time monitoring and response to the metrics.

As we considered the additional data requests for PAL-IS we determined that the data requirements were evolving from clinical to performance management requirements [22]. Business Intelligence (BI) is defined as a "set of methodologies, processes, architectures, and technologies that transform raw data into meaningful and useful information used to enable more effective strategic, tactical, and operational insights and decision-making" [23]. A BI application collects data to facilitate business process optimization in a flexible manner while enabling an organization to monitor and measure the performance of their business processes [24, 25]. These measurements are often used to identify how well a particular process is being performed [26]. To extend PAL-IS to support performance management we needed to develop a business intelligence (BI) application to enable monitoring of the community based processes. However, there are few methodological approaches for modeling a health system from the perspective of metrics, data sources, and process touch points to enable performance management of community based healthcare delivery. This paper addresses that shortcoming and presents a methodology for modeling goals, metrics and data to enable engineering of HIT to support performance management of community based care. Our paper has six sections. Sections 1 and 2 were the introduction and background to our research. Section 3 is our methodology for modeling goals, metrics and data to enable engineering of BI applications for performance management of community based care. Section 4 is proof of concept of our methodology using a case study from our palliative care research. Section 5 discussions the implications of our research. Section 6 is our conclusions.

3   Methodology

In this section we present a four step methodology for analyzing and modeling goals, metrics and data to enable engineering of BI applications for performance management of community based care. Figure 1 shows our overall methodology. Our methodology focuses on the lightweight development of BI applications that are easily deployed and which capture the minimum amount of data to compute the metrics required to provide insight into care process performance. Our methodology focuses on quick initial deployment of prototype BI applications that require small amounts of data to provide initial insights into performance of the care process. Subsequent versions of the BI application can be more comprehensive by refining and expanding the application model (and the data collected).

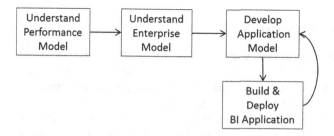

Fig. 1. Methodology for engineering of BI applications for community based care

3.1   Understand Performance Model

The performance model for a care process defines the goals for the care process and how they will be measured. For a community care process, the performance model might be quite complex. Regional authorities and accreditation agencies may have competing theories and models for the purpose of a care process and how it should be measured, while the participating organizations may have organizational goals that conflict. While the overall process may be to create a more efficient care delivery system, or to deliver patient centered care, the metrics and goals to measure performance may be varied and include clinical, service delivery and educational metrics and goals. However, it is not necessary to develop a complete and consistent performance model in order to build and deploy a BI application for measuring performance. Rather, it is important to understand who the key users and stakeholders for the BI application are; to identify where there is consensus on what the most important goals are; and to know what types of metrics could possibly be used to measure them. In this manner, a well-chosen simple subset of goals and metrics can be chosen to provide a BI application that provides useful (but not necessarily complete) visibility and insight into the performance of the care process.

3.2   Understand Enterprise Model

The enterprise model for a care process defines the information that is collected and shared for a process, including which resources collect or record the information and where they are located in the community. For a community care process, the enterprise model might be quite complex. Different organizations may have completely different approaches and HIT for managing their information related to the patient. Many organizations still use paper, faxes and phone calls. However, it is not necessary to develop a complete and consistent enterprise model of information in order to build and deploy a BI application for measuring performance. Rather, it is enough to understand which types of information and resources in the community, that are relevant to the metrics identified in Sect 3.1, might be the simplest to work with in order to provide the data needed by the BI application.

3.3   Develop Application Model

The next step in the methodology is to formally structure and model the insights gleaned from understanding the performance and enterprise model for the care process in an application model. This model will define the BI application as a minimal set of metrics that will give insight to a few of the more important goals, for which we can find resources in the community that will collect the minimal set of data attributes needed. In theory, this data could come as data feeds from HIT systems throughout the community. In practice, the data required is often not in electronic form (more often hybrid paper-electronic), or there are significant organizational barriers and processes that make it difficult to obtain the data in a timely fashion. In such situations, it is quicker and more effective to deploy mobile apps to appropriate care providers to enter the data in simple forms. Over time, with subsequent versions of the BI application, as the data needs are better understood, the mobile apps can be replaced with direct feeds from HIT systems.

Figure 2 shows the meta-model that we use as a basis for creating an application model for a BI application. The Care Process object names and describes the community care process linking it to performance goals for the process as well as resources across the community involved in the process. The Resource object represents touch points across the community care network (either care providers or HIT systems) where data can be collected. The Form object names a set of attributes that need to be collected at some point in the process in order to compute metrics. The Goal object describes outcomes expected to be achieved by the care process. The name uniquely identifies the goal. The description explains the meaning of the goal related to the performance of the care process. Goals can be decomposed into sub goals. The Metric object defines the measurement used to quantify a goal. It describes any computation that needs to be performed to measure the goal quantitatively.

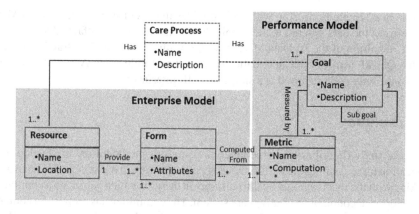

Fig. 2. Application meta-model

3.4 Build and Deploy BI Application

The final step of our methodology is to build and deploy a BI application based on the Application Model. This is diagrammed in Fig. 3. The Application Model defined in Sect. 3.3 identifies the Metrics to be evaluated and the Forms/Attributes which will be used to capture the data needed. To capture the Forms/Attributes a simple Mobile Form App is built. To store the data from the app and compute the necessary metrics a BI Data Mart is built from the Application model. The BI Data Mart uses a star-schema [27] in which Forms are stored in fact tables with relationships to lookup tables that specify the allowed values for Attributes. This structure allows flexible computation and reporting of metrics along different dimensions.

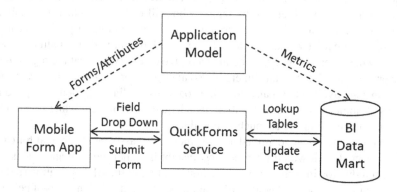

Fig. 3. Build and deploy BI application

We have built an open source middleware, QuickForms Service, which greatly simplifies the task of building such mobile apps and data marts in an integrated fashion. The QuickForms Service has an AJAX API, which links and populates the drop-down controls in a Mobile Form App with lookup-tables in the corresponding BI Data Mart. It then stores the data entered in the Mobile Form App as facts in a fact table.

The definition of the BI Data Mart from the Application model is straight forward, and the QuickForms Service automatically links the Mobile Form App to the BI Data Mart so the only code required is a simple HTML interface.

4 Case Study

This case study describes our experience in using our methodology to develop a BI application for measuring the performance of palliative care in our region. We have been working with the local regional health authority in our area which has set up a committee to develop an accountable palliative care system. The committee has proposed a comprehensive performance model. The local regional health authority also has a comprehensive enterprise model of resources and HIT in the region.

4.1 Performance Model

Since 2012 the regional Standards and Indicators Specialty Committee responsible for developing an accountable palliative care system has been meeting with the participation of approximately fifteen stakeholders from across the region. From fall 2012 to fall 2013 the committee developed a set of 22 metrics to support evidence based performance measurement of palliative care. These metrics are designed to give the committee a clear picture of palliative care in the region and can roughly be characterized in terms of three major goals: Access, Education and Care. The Access goal is to ensure that all palliative patients are identified in the region, and that all relevant palliative care services are available for them so that they receive appropriate treatment. The Education goal is to ensure that all care providers in the region who will come in contact with palliative patients have at least a basic level of training and understanding of palliative care and are aware of the palliative care services that are available for patients. Palliative care is a relatively new area of medicine and the palliative care services that the region is now able to provide are also new and emerging, so many care providers are not aware of the services that are available. Finally, the Care goal is for palliative patients to spend their last days at home, with pain and symptoms adequately managed, while remaining as conscious and enjoying life as much as possible.

For our case study, we identified a single metric and associated sub goal for each of these major goals that would give the most insight into their performance. This was a significant reduction in complexity for the first iteration of the BI Application (reducing from 22 metrics to 3 metrics) while still retaining significant value in terms of being able to provide insight into how well palliative care was being delivered in our region.

4.2 Enterprise Model

Our regional health authority comprises a group of 14 non-for-profit organizations that coordinates and funds delivery of health services in the Ontario community. The regional health authority coordinates services offered to the community in six main sectors: Hospitals, Community Care (nurses that provide at home care), Long Term Care (including retirement homes and hospices), Mental Health (including addiction services), Community Services (including social workers, pastoral care, meal services etc.), and Family Health (Family doctors and clinics).

Our case study aims to monitor palliative care across all six sectors. There is a diverse collection of HIT that is used in these sectors. In many cases, paper forms, faxes and phones are the only source of information. In other case where sophisticated HIT is in place (hospitals and some family health clinics) there are still significant technical, procedural and organizational barriers to collecting information in a common format across the region. As a result, the first iteration of our BI application focused in on the minimal set of data attributes that could be collected using a mobile form app.

It was generally believed that a significant majority of palliative patients eventually are visited at home by palliative care nurses in the community care sector. So they were identified as the key resource that could collect data for the metrics related to the Access and Care goals. For the metric related to the Education goal, the regional training administrator responsible for palliative care courses was identified as the key resource to collect data.

4.3   Develop Application Model

With a focused understanding of the relevant performance and enterprise models, we were now able to build an application model for our BI application. Figure 4 shows the application model. For each major goal we identified a single sub goal and metric to focus on, and linked it to a single resource in the community that would collect the data for that metric.

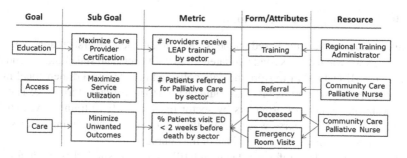

Fig. 4. Application model for palliative care

For education, the regional health authority is promoting a course called Learning Essential Approaches to Palliative Care (LEAP) [19], and it was decided to track how many providers by sector are receiving such training as the regional training administrator could easily provide those numbers. This can be done with a simple form app the administrator fills out each time the course is offered. In the long term, the region would like to track what percentage of care providers in each sector have received LEAP certification, but this would require interacting with all the organizations in each sector on an ongoing basis in order to get an accurate registry of the total number of care providers for all sectors and their certification status. For the first iteration, simply tracking the trend of numbers trained year by year for each sector will suffice.

For access, all palliative patients would benefit from a home care visit from a community care palliative nurse at some point. In the first iteration, it was decided to simply track how many patients are referred for such a service on a year to year basis by sector. This is easily done with a simple form app each time the nurse is assigned a new patient. In the long term, the region would like to identify palliative patients before they reach the stage where home care is needed. They would also like to track all the other palliative services the region provides. However, for the first iteration, this is the most critical service to track. There are specific complications associated with palliative patients that only a palliative nurse will be able to recognize and address. Without a home care visit, the likelihood of patient distress and unnecessary medical interventions increases.

For care, the most important sub goal is to minimize is unwanted outcomes. In particular, a palliative patient should be maintained comfortably at home during their last days with visits from a nurse and not require unexpected medical treatment that requires visiting an ER. Over the long term, it would be good to have on record every time a palliative patient visits the ER and whether this was accidental (e.g. falling and breaking a hip) or avoidable (i.e. insufficient pain management in the middle of the night). But obtaining this information is difficult as it would require changes to current ER procedures, and require integration with ER information systems. In addition, correlating such visits with patient death notices would be difficult. For the first iteration, it was decided that the palliative nurse would be the most likely resource able to record in a form app when a patient is deceased, and when they have had an ER visit.

4.4   Build and Deploy BI Application

To build the BI Application, based on the Application model, we first created mock-ups of the forms we wanted to use and validated them with users and stakeholders, and then we created a BI Data Mart to store the data collected in forms in a dimensional model that would flexibly support reports that could be used to measure performance. The form for tracking the number of providers by sector receiving LEAP training was straight forward. Every time a course was offered, the regional training administrator simply recorded the sector of each care provider in the course.

The forms for tracking referrals, deaths and ER visits were similarly straight forward. However, it was discovered that the community care palliative nurses already have a patient information form that records the referral date (which is request date on their form) and the deceased date for a patient. Rather than add a form for recording ER visits, it was decided for iteration 1 to simply add an attribute that indicated "Yes", "No", or "Not Known" if the patient had visited the ER in the last two weeks. The nurse would enter that information at the same time as entering the deceased date. Figure 5 shows a mock-up of the type of form that the palliative nurses are using.

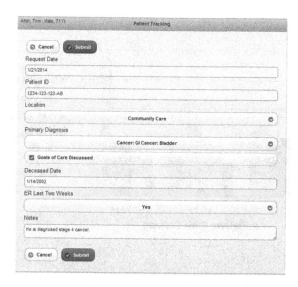

Fig. 5. Palliative patient information form

Once the forms for LEAP training and patient information were built in HTML, the forms and the attributes they collected were linked to the appropriate tables and columns in the database used by the BI Data Mart. With a fact table for training and a fact table for patient information, it was straight forward to define the metric computations and build three simple reports that would give insight on how the delivery of palliative care for the region was performing on a year by year basis. Sample mockups, that give an idea of how the reports will look, are shown on the next few pages. It should be emphasized that we are not showing actual data for 2012, 2013 and 2014 but rather we have created synthetic data that reflects the sort of results that the regional health authority would expect to see when they measure the performance of palliative care delivery once the BI application is deployed.

In Fig. 6, one can see at a glance whether or not the numbers of providers receiving training is increasing year over year. In particular, there is significant growth in the community service field. But with a closer look, one can also see that the numbers for long term care, mental health and family health while relatively steady, are dropping a little. This would probably prompt some follow up discussions with the different sectors. It is likely that the community service domain has a large and growing number of alternative providers (e.g. massage therapists, counsellors) that is fueling continued growth and it is possible that the Long Term Care sector has fully embraced LEAP so that it is only a small number of new care providers each year that need training. With respect to mental health and family health providers, though, it might be possible that they are too busy and are perhaps not seeing the value of the LEAP course. In discussions with those sectors the region might decide to tailor a course that more specifically meets their needs and offer it at more convenient times and locations.

In Fig. 7, one can see at a glance that referrals for palliative care service are growing across significantly across all sectors. This would be expected as the LEAP training is

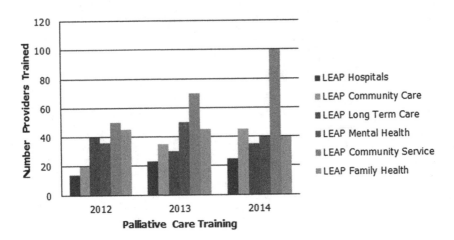

Number Providers Trained	LEAP					
	Hospitals	Community Care	Long Term Care	Mental Health	Community Service	Family Health
2012	14	20	40	36	50	45
2013	23	35	30	50	70	45
2014	25	45	35	40	100	40

Fig. 6. Number of providers receiving LEAP training

rolled out. The fact that no levelling off can be seen, would seem to indicate, though, that palliative care is still new and that not all the patients that should be receiving at home care from a community care palliative nurse are receiving it. Not surprising, the greatest growth is seen in the community care service where the nurses would be more aware of their colleagues that specialize in palliative care. One can also see an interesting anomaly in the data that might warrant further investigation where referrals from long term care went down in 2013 but bounced back in 2014.

Finally, in Fig. 8, one can see at a glance that the number of patients who visit the ER in the last two weeks of their life is trending down as you would hope would happen with an increase in LEAP training, and referrals for palliative nurses. At the same time, one can also see that roughly half of all patients are still ending up in the ER. There may be some systemic problems that need further investigation. For example, there may not be enough doctors and nurse practitioners available for home visits that can prescribe appropriate pain medication. One can also see at a glance that biggest improvement in numbers has been in the mental health sector. It can be tricky to get the right dose of pain medication for palliative care patients since delirium is often misdiagnosed as groans of pain when it is actually an indication that less pain medication is prescribed. This issue might have been compounded when mental health issues are present, but is now handled better with LEAP training and more referrals for palliative nurses.

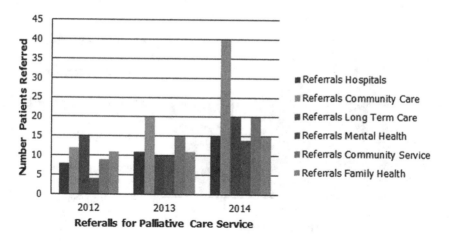

Number Patients Referred	Referrals					
	Hospitals	Community Care	Long Term Care	Mental Health	Community Service	Family Health
2012	8	12	15	4	9	11
2013	11	20	10	10	15	11
2014	15	40	20	14	20	15

Fig. 7. Number of patients referred for palliative care service

While we have not tested our method with actual data we have shown how it would work. The key implication from our method is that in a remarkably short time the regional health authority will be able to deploy a BI application that gives them insight into how well their palliative care processes are performing. Further, this is done with minimal effort and minimal disruption to the community resources that are providing care. It took two weeks of analysis to build the application model and only one week to build the BI application. Palliative care nurses have a single extra check box to fill in on their patient info form, and the regional training administrator has a single extra field to track (sector) for providers taking LEAP training.

The other important thing to note is that by zeroing in on the single most important metric for the three main goals (education, access, care), we have ended up with three simple reports that accurately capture the strategy of the region for improving delivery of palliative care. Namely, increased training and referrals for home care from palliative nurses should result in a reduction of unwanted outcomes (i.e. visits to ER).

5   Discussion

The paper introduced a methodology for modeling goals, metrics and data to enable engineering of business intelligence applications to support performance management of community based care. Our methodology makes several contributions to engineering

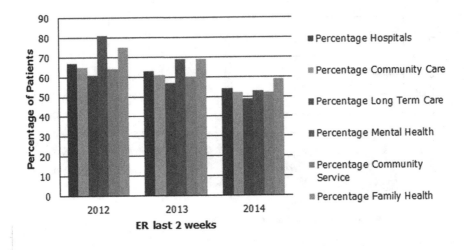

Percent of Patients	Percentage					
	Hospitals	Community Care	Long Term Care	Mental Health	Community Service	Family Health
2012	67	65	61	81	64	75
2013	63	61	57	69	60	69
2014	54	52	49	53	52	59

Fig. 8. Percentage of patients who visited the ER in the last 2 weeks of their life

business intelligence applications to support healthcare delivery. First, our method has a short implementation to analysis cycle to allow users to get rapid access to prototypes showing data analysis for monitoring performance. While the processes in the community are complex our objective was not to simplify them but rather to provide a simple and consistent way of reporting and monitoring performance. Second, our method minimizes the time and data entry effort required by the providers entering the data. Recognizing that it will likely be clinicians and managerial personnel entering the data we wanted to ensure that the system we designed was user friendly and not a burden. Third, as illustrated in the various proof of concept examples in Sect. 4.4, our approach provides the means to support decision making around relevant palliative care process issues such as referrals, training, and admissions to the ER. Currently these issues are disconnected from the data that would enable evidence based decision making about the issues. While our approach does not solve the issues per say, it does make it possible to collect data and provide metrics to support evidence based decision making. Monitoring metrics such as patient access to services and end-of-life admissions to the ER will support better patient outcomes and should ultimately lead to better quality end of life care.

Implementing performance management systems for community based care delivery is a challenge for several reasons. A particular challenge is that it requires the integration of data from several sources as patients have several data touch points throughout the community (e.g. family physician systems, ER departments, home care systems). To integrate data from all these systems would be an onerous task due to technical issues as well as organizational challenges and politics around data access permissions. Health IT system designers will typically only get once chance at designing an integrated application because of the complexity involved in integrating data from several systems and getting buy in from all the end users, which poses a risk in that the system requirements have little room for error. Our approach supports requirements engineering and systems design to identify and assess performance management through rapid prototypes so that outputs can be analyzed by end users to identify if changes are needed.

There are shortcomings to our approach. Foremost is we have not created a community based business intelligence HIT system but rather have developed a methodology to monitor metrics in the community. Therefore double entry will be required into the interface in our BI application (i.e. Fig. 5) and the HIT systems (e.g. electronic health records) that exist throughout the community. However, by mapping processes to goals, goals to metrics, and metrics to forms and data, (i.e. Fig. 2) we have identified the 'roadmap' for process monitoring in the community. Future work of ours will entail developing the integrated performance management system. Another shortcoming is the flexibility of our framework is achieved by a unified mobile design approach which has a trade-off of increased potential for erroneous data entry. Privacy issues are also a concern and will be dealt with in future iterations.

6 Conclusion

Monitoring care processes in the community is a challenge owing to the diversity of the processes and the variations in data that instantiates these processes. These process diversities and data variations make engineering business intelligence applications to monitor community processes difficult because of uncertainty in the system requirements. This paper presented a methodology for analyzing and modeling goals, metrics and data to enable engineering of BI applications for performance management of community based care. Our methodology helps identify the landscape of processes and data to enable identification of requirements and rapid development of BI applications that enables end users and decision makers to study outputs from the applications and change requirements if needed. As more care delivery is provided through diverse community settings methods such as our will play a key role in supporting evidence based healthcare delivery.

Acknowledgements. We acknowledge funding support from a Discovery Grant from the Natural Sciences and Engineering Research Council of Canada and a MITACS internship grant. We also thank the Champlain Hospice Palliative Care Program Standards and Indicators Specialty Committee, Champlain LHIN Community Care Access Centre, and Bruyere Continuing Care for their contributions to our research.

References

1. IOM (Institute of Medicine). Health IT and Patient Safety: Building Safer Systems For Better Care. The National Academies Press, Washington, DC (2012)
2. Kuperman, G.J., Bobb, A., Payne, T.H., Avery, A.J., Gandhi, T.K., Burns, G., Classen, D.C., Bates, D.W.: Medication-related clinical decision support in computerized provider order entry systems: a review. J. Am. Med. Inform. Assoc. **14**, 29–40 (2007)
3. Coiera, E.: Building a national health IT system from the middle out. J. Am. Med. Inform. Assoc. **16**(3), 271–273 (2009)
4. McKibbon, A., Lokker, C., Handler, S., Dolovich, L.R., Holbrook, A.M., O'Reilly, D., Tamblyn, R., Hemens, B.J., Basu, R., Troyan, S., Roshanov, P.S.: The effectiveness of integrated health information technologies across the phases of medication management: a systematic review. J. Am. Med. Inform. Assoc. **19**, 22–30 (2012)
5. Novak, L., Brooks, J., Gadd, C., Anders, S., Lorenzi, N.: Mediating the intersections of organizational routines during the introduction of a health IT system. Eur. J. Inf. Syst. **21**(5), 552–569 (2012)
6. Health IT in Long-term and post acute care. http://www.healthit.gov/sites/default/files/pdf/HIT_LTPAC_IssueBrief031513.pdf. Accessed Sep 2014
7. Harris, M.F., Chan, C.B., Dennis, S.M.: Coordination of care for patients with chronic disease (Editorial). Med. J. Aust. **191**, 85–86 (2009)
8. Bohmer, R.M.J.: The four habits of high-value health care organizations. New Eng. J. Med. **365**(22), 2045–2047 (2011)
9. Cornwell, J., Sonola, L., Levenson, R., Poteliakhoff, E.: Continuity of care for older hospital patients. The King's Fund (2012). www.kingsfund.org.uk/publications/continuity_of_care.html. Accessed Sep 2014
10. Reynolds, H.W., Sutherland, E.G.: A systematic approach to the planning, implementation, monitoring, and evaluation of integrated health services. BMC Health Serv. Res. **13**(1), 168 (2013)
11. Coiera, E.W., Aarts, J., Kulikowski, C.A.: The dangerous decade. J. Am. Med. Inform. Assoc. **19**(1), 2–5 (2012)
12. Hanson, R.: Good health information - an asset not a burden! Aust. Health Rev. **35**(1), 9–13 (2011)
13. Chukmaitov, A., Harless, D.W., Bazzoli, G.J., Carretta, H.J., Siangphoe, U.: Delivery system characteristics and their association with quality and costs of care: implications for accountable care organizations. Health Care Manage. Rev. **40**, 92–103 (2014)
14. Accreditation Canada. The value and impact of health care accreditation: a literature review (2014). www.accreditation.ca. Accessed Sep 2014
15. Coiera, E.: Why e-health is so hard. Med. J. Aust. **198**(4), 178–179 (2013)
16. Loeb, J.M.: The current state of performance measurement in health care. Int. J. Qual. Health Care **16**(Suppl 1), i5–i9 (2004)
17. World Health Organization Definition of Palliative Care. http://www.who.int/cancer/palliative/definition/en/. Accessed Sep 2014
18. Barbera, L., Paszat, L., Chartier, C.: Indicators of poor quality end-of-life cancer care in Ontario. J. Palliative Care **22**, 12–17 (2006)
19. Learning essential approaches to palliative and end-of-life care (LEAP). http://pallium.ca/more/learning-essential-approaches-to-palliative-and-end-of-life-care-leap/. Accessed 11 Sep 2014

20. Peyton, L., Kuziemsky, C. Langayan, D.: A case study in interoperable support for collaborative community healthcare. In: Proceedings of the 4th International Conference on Software Engineering in Health Care, pp. 8–14. IEEE Press (2012)

21. Baarah, A., Kuziemsky, C.E., Chamney, A., Bindra, J., Peyton, L.: A design strategy for health information systems to address care process management. In: Proceedings of the International Conference on Information and Communication Systems. IEEE Press (2014)

22. Baarah, A.: An Application Framework for Monitoring Care Processes, PhD Thesis, University of Ottawa, December 2013. https://www.ruor.uottawa.ca/handle/10393/30329. Accessed Sep 2014

23. Evelson, B.: Topic Overview: Business Intelligence. Forrester (2008)

24. Forrester Consulting. Enabling Dynamic Business Applications with BPM and SOA (2008)

25. Ko, R., Lee, S., Lee, E.: Business process management (BPM) standards: a survey. Bus. Process Manage. J. **15**(5), 744–791 (2009)

26. Kronz, A.: Managing of process key performance indicators as part of the ARIS methodology. In: Corporate Performance Management: ARIS in Practice, pp. 31–44. Springer, Heidelberg (2006)

27. Kimball, R., Ross, M.: The Data Warehouse Toolkit: The Complete Guide to Dimensional Modeling, 3rd edn. Wiley, New York (2013)

28. James, B.C.: Quality Management for Health Care Delivery. Hospital Research and Educational Trust, Chicago (1989)

29. Waterson, P.: Health information technology and sociotechnical systems: a progress report on recent developments within the UK National Health Service (NHS). Appl. Ergon. **45**(2 PA), 150–161 (2014)

Towards Continuous Certification of Clinical Information Systems

Jens H. Weber[1]([⊠]) and Craig Kuziemsky[2]

[1] Department of Computer Science,
University of Victoria, Victoria, BC, Canada
jens@uvic.ca
[2] Telfer School of Management, University of Ottawa, Ottawa, ON, Canada
Kuziemsky@telfer.uottawa.ca

Abstract. Clinical information systems (CISs) play an increasingly pivotal role in modern health care delivery. They are safety-critical as well as sensitive with respect to security and privacy concerns. In the light of ongoing reports on CISs failures and technology-induced adverse events, policy-makers and regulators have been struggling to identify effective ways to ensure the quality of these systems. Existing regulatory frameworks and controls do not readily apply to CISs. This paper identifies the shortcomings of existing regulatory controls and proposes a new framework for regulating CIS, based on a notion of *continuous* certification. We exemplify the application of the proposed framework with a real-world case study of a perioperative CIS.

Keywords: Clinical information system · Regulatory controls · Quality compliance · Certification · Interactions

1 Introduction

An Institute of Medicine report published in 2012 concluded that the present healthcare trajectory has become too complex and costly and that digital technology will be a key aspect of healthcare delivery [1]. Clinical Information systems (CISs) will play a critical role in helping health care authorities provide service delivery in the context of shrinking workforces and increased need for services [2, 3]. However there is a need for ways of evaluating and monitoring the quality of CIS implementation. To date the evidence base on the use and impact of CISs is limited and inconsistent. While studies have advocated positive outcomes from CISs [4], there is also a substantial body of research reporting on unintended outcomes including workflow, communication, and safety issues [5, 6]. Yet there is an overall dearth of frameworks that provide insight on these unintended outcomes to allow us to shape CIS certification to address the issues.

While there has been research on regulatory controls the complexity of the healthcare environments where CISs are used often limits the applicability of the controls. In the U.S. certification of specific types of CISs (i.e. electronic health records) is provided by the ONC Authorized Testing and Certification Bodies (ONC– ATCBs) while other types of CISs (e.g., picture archiving and communication systems - PACS) are licensed by the FDA [7]. However certification does not guarantee that CIS will actually be

© Springer International Publishing AG 2017
M. Huhn and L. Williams (Eds.): FHIES 2014/SEHC 2014, LNCS 9062, pp. 178–193, 2017.
DOI: 10.1007/978-3-319-63194-3_12

implemented and work as designed [8]. This is because clinical processes exist in a multi-agent environment that imposes external influences on how a CISs is used. Healthcare delivery is a complex environment of interactions [9] that must be considered as part of certification and regulatory compliance. However, understanding the interactive healthcare environment is challenging for several reasons. One is that the mixture of people, processes and technology must be viewed from a sociotechnical perspective [10]. Another reason is that the processes that are being automated through CISs are often abstract or incompletely defined, e.g., not all possible process deviations are considered. Moreover, collaborative healthcare delivery is a common objective of healthcare systems and therefore CIS are increasingly used to support collaborative activities. However, collaborative processes are immature and therefore in an evolving state [11].

The fundamental shortcoming in existing initiatives for CIS certification and regulatory compliance is that they are heavily focused on technological regulation, targeting concepts such as usability testing and interface design. A technology centered focus fails to consider the interactive sociotechnical environment where CISs is used. It is widely documented that regulators and healthcare administrators want quality assured CISs [12, 13]. However, traditional regulatory controls do not readily apply. This paper addresses that shortcoming and develops a new framework for regulating CISs that provides new perspectives on traditional notions of control. The framework has been developed from an engineering and management perspective. We use a case study of a perioperative CISs to articulate issues in CISs quality control and discuss how our framework addresses these issues.

The rest of this paper is structured as follows: The next section provides an overview on the regulator domains that are currently relevant to CISs. Section 3 presents foundational concepts and work related to certification of CISs. Section 4 describes a real world case study of a perioperative CISs. We present our continuous certification framework in Sect. 5 and exemplify its application with the perioperative case study in Sect. 6. We summarize our results and offer conclusions in Sect. 7.

2 Compliance and Quality of Clinical Information Systems

CISs are often critical with respect to safety as well as security and privacy. Moreover, the application of CISs is supposed to increase quality and efficiency of health care systems. Recognizing their sensitive nature, CISs are increasingly subject to regulation and standards, including mandatory, voluntary, and incentivised certification. In many jurisdictions, CIS related regulations and certification regimes have emerged from three traditionally separate "regulatory domains", namely (1) regulations on medical devices, (2) informational privacy and security laws, and (3) regulations on effective use of CIS.

The separation of these regulatory domains and their different approaches to compliance has been problematic, as the quality concerns they cover are overlapping. For example, safety and security concerns are intimately related when it comes to CISs and often consider the same factors, failure modes and effects. The only substantial difference between safety and security considerations consists of a difference of assumptions that underlie the threat analysis process: security analysis includes an assumption of possible malicious intent, while safety analysis (typically) does not. Moreover, in health care, the quality attribute of safety is intimately linked to that of effectiveness. Indeed, it has been argued that from a population health perspective it is sufficient to evaluate CIS installations with respect to performance (effectiveness) rather than including safety as another quality goal, as unsafe healthcare systems will naturally lead to less favourable health outcomes. Similar arguments (albeit less categorical) have been included in many medical devices regulations where residual safety risks are commonly weighed against the expected benefit of introducing medical devices.

2.1   Controls and Compliance

The three regulatory domains described above make use of significantly different controls to achieve compliance. Medical devices, including software-based devices such as CISs, often emphasize pre-deployment certification and licensing, followed by post-deployment surveillance, which is usually based on some type of "incident reporting system" [18]. Moreover, device-makers are usually required to attain process-based certification and licensing as a way to assure quality-manufacturing practices. In contrast, CIS related effectiveness and performance controls often emphasize post-deployment compliance measures, e.g., the U.S. and Canadian regulations on the "meaningful use" of healthcare IT [19]. The controls used to enforce security and privacy regulations are mainly based on legal obligations and penalties for violations of these obligations.

2.2   Criticism

Current regulatory frameworks and control models for CISs have been subject to much criticism. Pre-deployment certifications of CISs has been seen as ineffective and a threat to innovation. In contrast to traditional medical devices, software-based systems evolve frequently and many safety related concerns manifest only at or after deployment in the actual system environment [20]. In particular when it comes to CIS devices, safety concerns are often related to system customizations, the quality of the information content, and the organizational processes and workflows that surround the CIS use. Unfortunately, the controls currently available for post-deployment surveillance are very limited and largely deemed ineffective when it comes to CISs. While many jurisdictions operate incident reporting systems for (software) device users (e.g., the U.S. FDA's MAUDE), CIS-related reports submitted in these systems are rarely actionable and useful to improve on many of the hazards experienced with applying CIS in practice.

Moreover, CIS related incidents are assumed to be underreported, partially because they are difficult to detect and pin down, and partially because it is often difficult to decide who is at fault [1]. Since health information systems tend to be networked in large scale "systems of systems", the location of fault manifestation may be far away from to root cause of the error [20]. A further challenge to identifying the cause of CIS errors is the difficulty in defining the spaces within which CISs are used. Unlike technology designed for a closed environment (i.e. an airline cockpit, assembly line), CISs are often used in open systems, often referred to as 'spaces', which represent the interactive sociotechnical environment where CIS are used [3, 14]. The dynamic nature of these spaces makes it hard to pinpoint how a CIS will automate a task. A significant gap often exists between the ostensive (i.e. ideal representation depicted through flowcharts and models such as UML diagrams) and the performance (i.e. what actually takes place in real settings) dimensions of a task [15]. However, existing research on clinical spaces and CISs is limited in that much of the research is conceptual and simply describes the nature and challenges of these spaces. A better formalization of clinical spaces and the interactions within them would enable us to use them to guide quality control and compliance monitoring of CIS.

3 Foundations and Related Work

There has been consensus that CIS safety and security problems are of socio-technical nature [21]. Theories developed in the study of socio-technical systems (STS) suggest a paradigm shift, away from considering CISs as static *entities* (or devices), and towards considering them as dynamic *processes* [6]. Harrison's Interactive Sociotechnical Analysis (ISTA) framework is an influential example of this school of thought [6]. A related approach referred to as System-Theoretic Accident Model (STAMP) has been developed by Leveson for safety critical control systems [22]. In earlier work, we have adapted STAMP for the analysis of CISs [20]. This adapted model consists of a double control loop where a physician *perceives* and *controls* the patient's health process indirectly by interacting with a CIS. Other agents (such as nurses, pharmacists, laboratory technicians, etc., but also interoperable medical devices) are interacting with the CIS to carry out control actions and enter observations and measurements. The benefit of the control system model is a systematic categorization of classes of hazards that should be avoided or mitigated.

Communication between different actors (human or machine) is an important function of most CISs and safety incidents often relate to communication breakdowns. Coiera has developed fundamental work in this area, in particular his *Interaction Design Theory* seeks to introduce mathematical concepts in support of designing communication pathways [9]. He quantified the concept of *common ground* between actors in the health care space, which is important for effective communication and thus a safety relevant property. In earlier work, we extended this concept to consider CIS related technology factors and introduced it with the software engineering method *i** [23] in order to analyze safety properties of CISs [24].

Quality assurance in software engineering is often discussed in terms of two categories, namely *validation* and *verification* (V&V). The latter seeks to ensure that the software meets specified requirements (i.e., *"have we built the software right?"*), while the first asks the question whether the software meets the actual user needs (i.e., *"have we built the right software?"*) [33]. Certification methods have traditionally focused primarily on verification. While the use of formal methods for certification of CISs is still rare, testing is extensively used for assuring compliance with regulatory requirements.

As safety and security are properties of *systems* rather than products, their assurance requires both verification *and* validation. Originating in the nuclear and defense industry, Safety Case analysis has been proposed as a method to construct and reason about safety properties of a system [25]. The notion of safety cases has subsequently been generalized as Assurance Cases (AC) and applied to security arguments. More recently, regulated knowledge-industries (such as healthcare) have become interested in exploring the adoption of AC analysis as way to improve safety certification of products. However, current initiatives of investigating AC analysis concentrate on traditional, hardware-based medical devices, such as drug infusion pumps [26] and do not focus on CIS software, due to their size and complexity.

A common point of criticism of AC methodology is the lack of a formal semantics for interpreting the constructed arguments. Rushby suggests that a formalization of AC should combine logics for reasoning about arguments (verification) and epistemic knowledge to account for the developer's knowledge and reasoning about the environment (validation) [28]. The traditional way of "encoding" epistemic knowledge has been to build simulation models. However, the drawback of simulation models is that they tend to be too specific, making lots of implicit assumptions that may not hold true in reality. A better approach would draw epistemic knowledge from real world use of CISs systems. Controlled safety evaluation audits and usability experiments have been proposed as a means to validate systems in their deployment environment [29].

4   Case Study: Perioperative Information System

While the foundations of quality and continuous monitoring have been well defined, it is a challenge to do so for CISs. One of the significant challenges is the separation of operational aspects of CISs with the need for continuous monitoring. In Sect. 2.2 we introduced the notion of 'spaces' that refer to the boundaries within which CIS are used. Safety and other issues with CISs often occur after implementation due to interactions between various spaces within which HIT is used. These issues are often tacit or hidden errors in that they only emerge after a CIS has been implemented and used in practice [16].

Pre-deployment controls typically focus on four major artefacts - system requirements, software requirements, environmental assertions, and the actual implementation of the CIS software. Evaluation of these artefacts is typically done using a 'gold standard' that represents the desired output from a task. Quality control for biomedical technologies such as pacemakers blood glucose monitors, or blood glucose measures have gold standards (i.e. systolic and diastolic blood pressure reading) that is the basis for evaluation and quality criteria. Therefore it can be easily identified when these technologies fail to meet appropriate values. However, the monitoring of CISs is a challenge because the nature of the various interactions (i.e. user, policy, clinical) within the spaces they are used. From the four categories of artefacts described above we believe the environmental assertion and actual implementations are the biggest challenges to quality control and compliance monitoring because they will vary by circumstances defined by the spaces where they are used. Smith and Koppel describe 45 scenarios within five overarching categories of CISs facilitated implementation problems that range from issues with data granularity to process and workflow issues [17].

Given the variation and complexity of the different spaces where CISs are used we believe the spaces need to be formalized and incorporated into quality compliance frameworks. In this section we present a new framework for regulating CIS that provides new perspectives on traditional notions of control. We use a perioperative case study to define categories of spaces implications.

One of the authors (CK) conducted a study of a perioperative CIS called the Surgical Information Management System (SIMS). SIMS was implemented in April 2009 in a multi-campus hospital in an urban Canadian City across all perioperative areas (pre-admit unit (PAU), same day admit (SDA), surgical day care (SDC), operating room (OR) and post-anaesthesia care unit (PACU)). The goal of SIMs was to bring common data and connectivity across the perioperative spectrum to promote collaboration and patient safety. From April 2012 to June 2013 he conducted over 130 h of non-participant observations across all the perioperative areas and campuses. He also conducted 8 interviews and 3 focus groups with different categories of users including anaesthetists, nurses and managers. The observations were transcribed to identify processes, agents and data sources pertaining to tasks both within and across the perioperative areas. The purpose of the study was to study how SIMS facilitated collaboration and coordination across the perioperative spectrum [34]. We have re-analyzed the data and findings from that study to study the overall 'space' where SIMS was used in order to identify the interactions within the space that impact quality and compliance monitoring.

From our case study we identified four categories of interactions that were facilitators of quality issues: data, knowledge, inferences and interoperability. The categories refer to interactions included interoperability of modules within SIMS, data checks and consistency, interoperability with other CIS systems (i.e. PACS or EHR systems) and how the software design (i.e. drop down lists or menus) supports specific clinical tasks (i.e. data entry, retrieval or decision making).

Data interactions include the entry and retrieval of data. For example, nurses described how a common challenge was how to find the correct field to enter data because of the number of menus and data entry options. A workaround to that problem was to put the data into a memo box. However that could cause safety or coordination issues as other providers may not always look in memo boxes and therefore important data could be missed.

Knowledge interactions refer to the integration of different data fields to support a task. For example, patients in the operating room often receive complex cocktails of anaesthesia drugs that involve three or four drugs of different percentages. Prior to SIMS the cocktails were written out by hand. In SIMS the drugs are selected by a drop down menu listing the different drug cocktails. During observations anaesthetists pointed out that the integrated drug list was cognitively taxing for decision making because many of the cocktails had similar drug names. The similar names combined with multiple drug concentration percentages provide opportunities for entry errors.

Interoperability interactions refer to cross-area interoperability of SIMS. For example, patients in the OR often receive prophylactic antibiotics to prevent infection after surgery. OR nurses were documenting the prophylactic antibiotics in a specific section of the *OR Manager* module of SIMS. However the issue is that the SIMS module in each perioperative area was not always interoperable across other areas. Specifically, the *OR Manager* module does not integrate with the module used in the next perioperative area (PACU). So while RNs in PACU could see what medications anaesthetists gave in the OR (because the document in the *Anaesthesia Manager* module which is interoperable with PACU), they could not see what medications RNs were giving in the OR. As a result PACU nurses had no idea that prophylactic antibiotics were being given to patients in the OR.

Inference interactions refer to decision support or care pathways that have been designed to guide care delivery. Examples include where a set protocol is used to support handoffs and other transitional tasks. For example, when an operation is completed and the anaesthetist goes to transfer the patient from the OR to PACU they receive a checklist of tasks (e.g. transfer patient with oxygen) to ensure an efficient and safe transfer takes place.

A final interaction consideration from our case study is the temporal aspect of how interactions evolve. As discussed in Sect. 1 a significant challenge with healthcare delivery is process immaturity. While there were certain tasks or design objectives that SIMS was engineered to achieve, the processes conducted by the clinicians often lacked maturity. The complex nature of healthcare delivery implies that we cannot always predict how interactions between CISs and people and processes will occur. As processes mature and evolve the evaluation metric may change and will alter how SIMS needs to be assessed. Further in-situ use of a CIS may identify new safety or quality issues that need to be incorporated into quality control and compliance monitoring. Therefore certification must include effective post-deployment controls as well as pre-deployment assurances. We will describe a framework for such controls in the next section and then illustrate its application to our case study in Sect. 6.

5   Continuous Regulation and Quality Control

5.1   Pre-deployment Controls

Figure 1 summarizes the continuous certification process for CISs proposed in this paper. The upper part of the figure depicts activities related to pre-deployment controls, while the lower part concerns post-deployment controls (surveillance).

Pre-deployment controls revolve around three major arguments (marked as checkpoints in the depicted process) and four major artefacts, i.e., system requirements, software requirements, environmental assertions, and the actual implementation of the CIS software device.

As in most other cyber-physical system domains, the distinction between system requirements and software requirements is of key importance. Clearly, CISs consist of software, as well as hardware, data, human operators and other factors. However, the focus of our process is on *software* certification. We therefore consider any system component that is not represented in software as part of the software device's *environment*. As a consequence of this viewpoint, we do not directly consider the design, implementation, and evolution such environmental components. Rather, we restrict ourselves to making assertions about these environmental components (and to validating whether these assertions agree with reality). This viewpoint is in line with current regulatory frameworks for certifying medical devices, which attempt to reason about safety and effectiveness of devices in context of their *intended* use environments. An important difference compared to traditional medical devices certification frameworks is, however, that we do not explicitly consider pre-*market* certification and controls in our model. Pre-*market* certification (in contrast to pre-*deployment* certification) does not consider the particular systems context of the client side where the CIS is being deployed. The rationale for this decision is the fact that CIS (in contrast to traditionally medical devices) tend to be heavily customized and adapted in order to fit their individual deployment system requirements.

In our model (Fig. 1), this viewpoint is reflected in the fact that each system requirement must either be *discharged* by requirements on the software or *addressed* by an environmental assertion. (The latter may give rise to a non-software requirement that must be discharged by non-software means, e.g., operator training, hardware design, space layout, etc.) Verifying that each system requirement is covered either by software behaviour or by environmental constraints is one of the three arguments (*completeness*) to be checked pre-deployment.

A second argument to be verified during pre-deployment evaluation concerns the *correctness* of the software device's implementation with respect to the specified software requirements. Different techniques may be used to gather evidence supporting

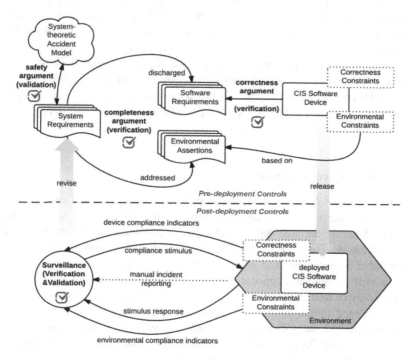

Fig. 1. Continuous certification process for clinical information systems

this argument, including but not limited to formal method proofs, static and dynamic code analysis, testing, etc.

The third argument to be checked concerns *safety* and validates the system requirements against a system-theoretic accident model for safety-critical information systems. The accident model provides a classification of different categories of hazards pertaining to CIS and can thus be used to systematically probe for potential safety threats. Threats are identified based on an additional set of system requirements and their mitigation may give rise to further system requirements. Validation of the pre-deployment safety validation argument requires that all hazards in the accident model be addressed by system requirements. As described above, each system requirement in turn may either be discharged by software (i.e., it gives rise to a software requirement) or it may be balanced by an assertion about the rest of the system (the software environment).

Following this model, safety accidents may arise as a result of one of three different types of failures: (1) failure to identify all safety-relevant system requirements, (2) failure to correctly implement a software requirement that discharges a safety-relevant system requirement, or (3) failure to make valid assertions about the environment of the software device. Reported evidence on accidents with CISs indicates that relatively few incidents are caused by type 2 failures [18]. Indeed, type 1 and 3 failures are "*validation*" failures as opposed to "*verification*" failures and thus difficult to detect outside the actual deployment environment. They are a primary reason for putting in place post-deployment controls. Existing post-deployment controls for CISs (which are mainly based on manual incident reporting) are not very effective, however, as described earlier. Our approach therefore focuses on the formal definition of constraints that can be evaluated automatically by a software device in operation. We consider *correctness constraints* that verify software correctness as well as *environmental constraints* to validate environmental assertions. Correctness constraints are akin to the well-known concept of design-by-contract in software engineering, while environmental constraints probe the software environment and thus can be seen as "environmental contracts". The concept of environmental constraints is new and we will provide examples later in this paper.

5.2   Post-deployment Controls

Once a CIS software device is deployed as part of a concrete system environment, it can be expected that the entire system will dynamically evolving over time. The lower part of Fig. 1 shows the post-deployment controls proposed in our continuous certification framework. They supplement the classical manual incident reporting process with a number of pro-active and automated compliance reports that encompass verification as well as validation concerns. Specifically, automated compliance reports are based on two mechanisms (1) compliance indicators, which are based on evaluating the previously defined formal correctness constraints and environmental constraints, and (2) an evaluation of the CIS response to given compliance stimuli (which can be considered deployed CIS test cases). We will discuss examples for such compliance stimuli and compliance indicators in the next section.

Figure 1 shows that the results of monitoring compliance indicators and responses to compliance stimuli (as well as manual incident reports) are used to inform the next revision of the system requirements, the software requirements, the device implementation, and the assertions made about the device environment. This feedback is in line with common quality management processes such as ISO 13485 (Quality management for medical devices) and the more general ISO 9001 standard on software quality management. Of course, the monitoring results may also be used to invoke changes to the environment of the software device, e.g., change organization procedures, training procedures, etc.

Notably, in the above discussion we did not prescribe which entity should own the post-deployment surveillance process. Three main possibilities present themselves, namely the regulator, the device manufacturer, and the device user (i.e., the system operator). All three scenarios are possible and can potentially be combined. For example, the device manufacturer may own the process that monitors device compliance indicators (i.e., software correctness concerns), the system operator may own the process that monitors environmental compliance indicators, and the regulator may own the process that monitors responses to compliance stimuli. What is ultimately important from a certification perspective is that all three processes are put in place.

6 Framework Applied to Case Study

In this section we will draw on our perioperative CIS case study described in Sect. 4 to illustrate the application of the continuous certification framework presented in the previous section.

6.1 Pre-deployment Controls

As described in the previous section, pre-deployment controls hinge on three main claims, a safety argument, a completeness argument and a correctness argument.

The **safety argument** is based on an analysis of the system requirements relative to a system-theoretic accident model. System requirements can be captured with a variety of different methods, e.g., goal-based models, agent activity models, use case maps, etc. Our certification framework does not prescribe a particular method for capturing system requirements. For the purpose of this paper, we will denote example requirements in natural language, in order to keep our presentation simple. In particular, we consider the following example requirements to illustrate the framework:[1]

- R1: Anaesthetists prescribe analgesic medication for patients prior to surgery.
- R2: Nurses and anaesthetists may administer analgesic medication.
- R3: The administration of analgesic medication must be documented and communicated to all clinicians in the perioperative circle of care of a patient.

---

[1] We use these requirements to illustrate our framework. Of course, the complete set of system requirements as documented in our case study system is more extensive.

Using a system-theoretic accident model (such as STAMP) to analyze the system requirements will reveal potential system-related hazards that must be addressed during pre-deployment certification. In the case of STAMP, the system is modelled as a controlled process loop, where the anaesthetist is seen as the controlling agent, the patient's surgical care is seen as the controlled process, and nurses (as well as anaesthetists) are seen as actuators that execute control actions (i.e., administer medications). The accident model defines a taxonomy of possible hazards that need to be addressed in the CIS safety argument. Two examples are *"disturbance and inappropriate control actions"* and *"delayed or missing feedback of control actions"*. Clearly, it is important from a safety perspective to inform anaesthetists as well as other clinicians in the patient's circle of care about control actions undertaken (i.e. administration of medication) in a reliable and timely manner in order to minimize adverse interoperability interactions. The definition of a safety claim with respect to this hazard may give rise to additional system requirements such as:

- R4: Administered medication is documented and communicated to the circle of care immediately.
- R5: Clinicians check for update of medication administration record directly before any medication administration action.

The **completeness argument** requires the software implementer to verify that all system requirements are either discharged to software requirements or addressed by assumptions on the system environment for deploying the software, or a combination of both. For example, the above requirements may give rise to a software requirement (SR1) *and* an environmental assertion (EA1), as presented below:

- SR1: Medication administration actions documented in SIMS are immediately communicated to all SIMS software components, and relevant connected system components
- EA1: Reliable access to the SIMS is provided at or near the point of care where analgesic medications are administered and caregivers use the software to log drug administration directly after the action was taken.

The **correctness argument** requires assurances for the correct implementation of software requirements. These assurances can be generated using a variety of verification methods as described earlier. We note, however, that CIS components are often subject to composition and customization at the deployment site (*after* release of the software). The assurance provided by pre-deployment correctness verification is therefore limited a particular system configuration under test. It is therefore important to define correctness constraints and environmental constraints that can be monitored post-deployment.

6.2   Post-deployment Controls

An example for correctness constraints guarding the interoperability of a software system after deployment is presented below. (Again, we use natural language to simplify presentation in this paper.)

- CC1: The entry of a medication order **o** for a patient **p** will eventually result in _exactly_ one documented action of substance administration **a** for order **o′** for patient **p′** where **p** = **p′** and **o** = **o′** and **a** ≈ **o**.

The constraint checks whether the data provided in the control order is unmarred and identical with the data used for executing the action (**o** and **p**) and whether the actual action taken **a** is equivalent to the prescribed order **o**. (The actual action taken may not always be identical with the prescribed order. For example, different drugs may be available as prescriptions may refer to generic substances while administration logs may refer to brand names etc.)

In practice, CC1 could be implemented at the interoperability interface of the SIMS system component that provides the prescription order entry functionality (_Anaesthesia Manager_). It expects connecting software components (such as the PACU OR Manager) to 'round-trip' the order data (**p** and **o**) along with the actual log of the administered action (**a**). Correctness constraint CC1 would be effective in catching several of the problems discussed in our case study. Specifically, it would detect data interaction issues related to nurses not using the right input form for entering data (**a** ≈ **o** would be violated) and data interoperability issues related to a configured system components that do not properly process orders (**p** = **p′** or **o** = **o′** would be violated).

Notably, CC1 does not yet address the aspect of timeliness of feedback to control actions. As described above, the timeliness aspect is partially discharged by software and partially based on an environmental assumption. We can add a correctness constraint to take account of this concern from a software-centric point of view:

- CC2: A substance administration action logged at time **t** must be received at time **t′** by all relevant SIMS components, with $\mathbf{t'} - \mathbf{t} < \Delta_I$

Similarly, we can define an environmental concern to assert assumptions about the software environment:

- EA2: A substance administration action taken at time **k** must be logged at time **k′** with $\mathbf{k'} - \mathbf{k} < \Delta_a$

During post-deployment CIS surveillance, data on violations to either correctness constraints or environmental constraints are continuously collected and monitored as device or environmental compliance indicators, respectively (see Fig. 1).

6.3   Using Compliance Stimuli/Responses for Assuring Knowledge Interaction

While the above approach of encoding constraints can be effective in addressing safety issues related to data interactions and interoperability, it is not well suited for addressing knowledge interactions and inference interactions (as defined in our case study). Our continuous certification framework addresses these kinds of issues with a compliance _stimulus/response_ model. We propose that any CIS that incorporates a knowledge-base (e.g., a decision support system) or that is used in support of complex cognitive functions performed by clinicians should incorporate a mechanism to process so-called "compliance stimuli". This idea is not new but is based on earlier work in context of continuously assuring safety of decision support systems in the Leapfrog project [30]. Essentially, the concept of compliance stimuli is akin to that of realistic test cases that may be submitted to the CIS under surveillance. These test cases are designed to trigger certain knowledge interactions or inferences and the resulting responses are compared against certain expected characteristics.

This process may be fully automated or manual, depending on the function to be tested. For example, the inference functions of a decision support system to trigger alerts based on drug-drug interactions or drug-allergy interactions may be tested automatically, while a software-based prescribing system will include manual (human) intervention in responding to compliance stimuli. Compliance indicators collected in this stimulus/response model are useful in detecting hazards and hazardous trends related to knowledge bases and cognitive functions. We believe that these methods will be sensitive for detecting the kind of knowledge and inference interaction issues observed in our case study. For example, the checklist that anaesthetists receive before transferring a patient from the OR to PACU can be verified by checking if an anaesthetist has responded to the checklist. Similarly the selection of anaesthesia medication from the complex dropdown list can be checked against the historical record of the anaesthetist for similar surgical procedures. Excessive variations in drugs, doses or concentrations can be flagged to the anaesthetist to verify if the current selection is indeed correct. It is important to point out that the compliance stimulus does not necessarily need to rely on technical specifics of a particular system deployment, but may rather use common information and knowledge interchange formats, as discussed in [31, 32].

7 Summary and Conclusions

As CIS become a larger part of healthcare delivery there is a need to monitor them with respect to quality control and regulatory compliance. While frameworks exist for regulatory compliance and quality control the sociotechnical complexity of healthcare delivery makes it difficult to use these frameworks. This paper has attempted to address that issue by proposing a new framework for regulating CISs, based on a notion of *continuous* certification. A common finding from existing research on CISs is that there is often a difference between how CISs are designed and how they are actually used in real clinical 'spaces'. Clinical spaces introduce boundaries and facilitate interactions between people, processes and technology that influence how a CIS is used. Further actual CIS usage often differs from the ostensive representation depicted through flowcharts or use cases. While research exists on clinical spaces and interactions, and has acknowledged the role they play in influencing CIS usage, much of the existing research is conceptual and does not provide guidance on how to better engineer and monitor CIS quality.

To compensate for that issue our framework ties together pre and post deployment controls into a continuous certification process. Pre-deployment controls focus on the major artefacts of a CIS (i.e. system environment and software components) and their safety properties with respect to a general accident model. It provides a boundary the clinical space to monitor quality and compliance of a CIS. Post-deployment controls focus on quality and compliance monitoring once a system has been implemented in a clinical setting. It focuses on the dynamic and at times evolving nature of the clinical space. We also used a case study of a perioperative CIS to develop a set of software and system requirements and environmental assertions for pre-deployment controls, and a set of constraints and concerns for post-deployment controls. The various requirements and constraints we developed help to formalize the clinical space and the interactions that occur within the space. While it is not possible to predict all the interactions and process evolution that co-exist with CIS usage our framework does provide a starting point for defining clinical spaces and interactions as part of compliance monitoring and quality regulation.

Limitations of our work are that we have only evaluated our framework using one case study of a very specific CIS. Other system requirements, environmental assertions, constraints and concerns may arise from other types of CISs (e.g. order entry systems) and settings.

Acknowledgements. We acknowledge funding support from the Natural Sciences and Engineering Research Council of Canada.

References

1. IOM (Institute of Medicine). Health IT and Patient Safety: Building Safer Systems For Better Care. The National Academies Press, Washington, DC (2012)
2. Kuperman, G.J., Bobb, A., Payne, T.H., Avery, A.J., Gandhi, T.K., Burns, G., Classen, D. C., Bates, D.W.: Medication-related clinical decision support in computerized provider order entry systems: a review. J. Am. Med. Inform. Assoc. **14**, 29–40 (2007)
3. Coiera, E.: Building a national health IT system from the middle out. J. Am. Med. Inform. Assoc. **16**(3), 271–273 (2009)
4. McKibbon, A., Lokker, C., Handler, S., Dolovich, L.R., Holbrook, A.M., O'Reilly, D., Tamblyn, R., Hemens, B.J., Basu, R., Troyan, S., Roshanov, P.S.: The effectiveness of integrated health information technologies across the phases of medication management: a systematic review. J. Am. Med. Inform. Assoc. **19**, 22–30 (2012)
5. Ash, J.S., Berg, M., Coiera, E.: Some unintended consequences of information technology in health care: the nature of patient care information system-related error. J. Am. Med. Inform. Assoc. **11**, 104–112 (2004)
6. Harrison, M.I., Koppel, R., Bar-Lev, S.: Unintended consequences of information technologies in health care: an interactive socio technical analysis. J. Am. Med. Inform. Assoc. **14**, 542–549 (2007)
7. Health Information Technology: Revisions to initial set of standards, implementation specifications, and certification criteria for electronic health record technology federal register (2011). http://edocket.access.gpo.gov/2010/pdf/2010-25683.pdf. Accessed 11 Apr 2014
8. Singh, H., Classen, D.C., Sittig, D.F.: Creating an oversight infrastructure for electronic health record-related patient safety hazards. J. Patient Saf. **7**(4), 169–174 (2011)
9. Coiera, E.: Interaction design theory. Int. J. Med. Inform. **69**, 205–222 (2003)

10. Weber-Jahnke, J.H., Price, M., Williams, J.: Software engineering in health care, is it really different? And How to gain impact. In: Proceedings of the 5th International Conference on Software Engineering in Health Care, pp. 1–4. IEEE press (2013)
11. Reddy, M.C., Gorman, P., Bardram, J.: Special issue on supporting collaboration in healthcare settings: the role of informatics. Int. J. Med. Inform. **80**(8), 541–543 (2011)
12. Sittig, D.F., Classen, D.C.: Safe electronic health record use requires a comprehensive monitoring and evaluation framework. JAMA **303**, 450–451 (2010)
13. Koppel, R.: Monitoring and evaluating the use of electronic health records. JAMA **303**, 1918–1919 (2010)
14. Coiera, E.: Communication spaces. JAMIA **21**(3), 414–422 (2014)
15. Novak, L., Brooks, J., Gadd, C., Anders, S., Lorenzi, N.: Mediating the intersections of organizational routines during the introduction of a health IT system. Eur. J. Inf. Syst. **21**, 552–569 (2012)
16. Coiera, E., Aarts, J., Kulkowski, C.: The dangerous decade. J. Am. Med. Inform. Assoc. **19**, 2–5 (2012)
17. Smith, S.W., Koppel, R.: Healthcare information technology's relativity problems: a typology of how patients' physical reality, clinicians' mental models, and healthcare information technology differ. J. Am. Med. Inform. Assoc. **21**, 117–131 (2014)
18. Weber-Jahnke, J.H.: A preliminary study of apparent causes and outcomes of reported failures with patient management software. In: Proceedings of 3rd International Workshop on Software Engineering in Health Care (SEHC), Co-Located with ICSE. ACM Press (2011)
19. Hogan, S.O., Kissam, S.M.: Measuring meaningful use. Health Aff. **29**(4), 601–606 (2010)
20. Weber-Jahnke, Jens H., Mason-Blakley, F.: On the safety of electronic medical records. In: Liu, Z., Wassyng, A. (eds.) FHIES 2011. LNCS, vol. 7151, pp. 177–194. Springer, Heidelberg (2012). doi:10.1007/978-3-642-32355-3_11
21. Leviss, J.: HIT or Miss: Lessons Learned from Health Information Technology Implementations. AHIMA Press, Chicago (2013). ISBN #:9781584263975
22. Leveson, N.: Engineering a Safer World: Systems Thinking Applied to Safety. MIT Press, Cambridge (2011)
23. Yu, E.S.K.: Social Modeling for Requirements Engineering. MIT Press, Cambridge (2011)
24. Kuziemsky, C.E., Weber-Jahnke, J., Williams, J.: Engineering the healthcare collaboration space. In: 4th International Workshop on Software Engineering in Health Care (SEHC), pp. 51 –57 (2012)
25. Cofer, D., Hatcliff, J., Huhn, M., Lawford, M.: Software certification: methods and tools (Dagstuhl Seminar 13051). Dagstuhl Reports **3**(1), 111–148 (2013)
26. Bloomfield, R., Bishop, P.: Safety and assurance cases: past, present and possible future – an adelard perspective. In: Dale, C., Anderson, T. (eds.) Making Systems Safer, pp. 51–67. Springer, London (2010)
27. Rushby, J.: Formalism in safety cases. In: Dale, C., Anderson, T. (eds.) Making Systems Safer. Springer, London (2010)
28. Borycki, E., et al.: Usability methods for ensuring health information technology safety: evidence-based approaches. contribution of the IMIA working group health informatics for patient safety. Yearb. Med. Inform. **8**(1), 20–27 (2013)
29. Kilbridge, P.M., Welebob, E.M., Classen, D.C.: Development of the Leapfrog methodology for evaluating hospital implemented inpatient computerized physician order entry systems. Qual. Saf. Health Care **15**, 81–84 (2006)

30. Bilykh, I., Jahnke, J.H., McCallum, G., Price, M.: Using the clinical document architecture as open data exchange format for interfacing EMRs with clinical decision support systems. In: Proceedings of IEEE International Conference on Computer Based Medical Systems - CBMS 2006, pp. 855–860 (2006)
31. Weber-Jahnke, J.H.: Design of decoupled clinical decision support for service-oriented architectures. Int. J. Software Eng. Knowl. Eng. 19(2), 159–183 (2009)
32. Boehm, B.W. (ed.): Software Risk Management. IEEE Press, Piscataway (1989)
33. Kuziemsky, C.E., Bush, P.: Coordination considerations of health information technology. Stud. Health Technol. Inform. 194, 133–138 (2013)

Applying Information System Hazard Analysis to an Episodic Document Context

Fieran Mason-Blakley(✉), Jens Weber, Abdul Roudsari, and Morgan Price

University of Victoria, 3800 Finnerty Road, Victoria, BC, Canada
fmason@uvic.ca
http://www.uvic.ca

Abstract. In spite of wide spread knowledge in the Clinical Information Technology (CIT) community about the unintended and sometimes hazardous consequences of the implementation and use of this technology, the application of systematic hazard analysis techniques in the domain for implementation projects, change management operations, or even prospective or retrospective static analysis have been sparsely reported. We report on the application of the Information Systems Hazard Analysis (ISHA) process to a conceptual architecture based on implementations of an electronic medical document exchange standard which was recently prescribed in British Columbia, Canada. The application of the technique with a focus on control coordination hazards identified a number of well known CIT hazards as well as a variety of less known hazards which the context presents.

Keywords: Health information technology · Risk assessment · Hazard analysis · Safety · Integrity

1 Introduction

In her 1999 report, Kohn reported that between 44000 and 98000 Americans die each year as a result of medical error. Kohn also showed that in spite of early indications, health information technologies (HIT) (a super-set of clinical information technologies (CITs)), had not delivered on their promise to reduce the number or severity of medical error; rather, these tools had been implicated as the source of a variety of new medical errors [20]. Clancy [9] and Bogner [4] followed up on Kohn's work ten years later. Neither found that the situation had improved, and in fact, Clancy found that it had worsened.

A number of researchers have studied the nature of these new errors including Koppel, Ash, Coiera and Aarts. In [21] Koppel discusses mechanisms by which CIT facilitates medical errors directly, while in [22] he describes how workarounds which arise to account for misalignment between CIT and workflow present risks of medical error. Ash discusses similar topics in her work. In [2] she discusses how consequences of CIT implementation tend to be pervasive and challenging to qualify. Some consequences will be intentional while others may be unintentional.

© Springer International Publishing AG 2017
M. Huhn and L. Williams (Eds.): FHIES 2014/SEHC 2014, LNCS 9062, pp. 194–213, 2017.
DOI: 10.1007/978-3-319-63194-3_13

Some of these intentional and unintentional consequences may be either universally desirable or undesirable. Others may or may not be desirable based on ones perspective. In [3], Ash discusses the prevalence of unintended consequences of computerized provider order entry (CPOE) (a specific type of CIT) across 176 US hospitals based on the results of a telephone survey. Coiera and Aarts warn in [10] that we are at risk of perpetuating the situations described by Kohn, Bogner and Clancy over the next ten years when more CIT will be deployed than in the entirety of the history of medicine. They suggest that though the relative rate of patient harm resulting from these technologies may remain constant, their prevalence will lead to an absolute increase in patient harm unless the issues which lead to dangers with these tools are addressed. Koppel, Ash, Coiera, Aarts and many others have begun investigation into the risks which CIT can present, but they do not employ systematic risk assessment techniques in their investigations. The sociotechnical methods they employ provide valuable insight, but techniques specifically designed to uncover hazards may be better suited to the task of analyzing the dangers presented by these technologies.

In safety critical industries like nuclear power and aviation, the application of hazard analysis and safety oriented design are common place [23]. Even in the general field of health care, application of retrospective techniques has been common for some time [13]. Recently however, the prescription of annual prospective safety analyses for accreditation by both the Joint Commission on the Accreditation of Healthcare Organizations (JCAHO) and by Accreditation Canada [15] has lead to an increased need for an understanding of available methodologies.

In spite of this increased focus, the application of these methods is sparsely reported as extending to, or including the CIT software devices which are increasingly central to the process of health care [8]. In fact, only a few applications of risk analysis techniques to these technologies could be uncovered in the literature. Win [32] and Bonnabry [5–7] leverage the failure modes and effects criticality analysis (FMECA) methodology on various CIT systems while Weber [31] applies a variety of retrospective systematic hazard analysis techniques to a combination of MAUDE (an FDA database of medical device related adverse events) reports and to an adverse event reported by Horsky [18].

In our present work, we report the application of the Information Systems Hazard Analysis (ISHA) process [24] to a conceptual architecture for an implementation of the recently prescribed, HL7 (Health Level 7) V3 CDA (Clinical Document Architecture) [12] based, Electronic Medical Record (EMR) to Electronic Medical Record (E2E) exchange standard [16]. The architecture is a generalization of the designs of a number of systems which support this standard. E2E addresses four primary clinical processes: EMR exchange, patient export, episodic document exchange and finally unstructured document exchange. As ISHA has a strong focus on coordination of control, we analyze the episodic document business context where these strengths of the method provide the most value.

The rest of this article is composed of three additional sections. In Sect. 2, background, we discuss the theoretical and process basis of ISHA. We then proceed to introduce the ISHA method and its steps and some work related to the method. We finish the background section by introducing the E2E standard paying specific attention to the episodic document context. In Sect. 3, analysis, we apply the ISHA method in stepwise fashion to the E2E episodic document use case. Finally, in Sect. 4, conclusions and current work, we summarize the results of our investigation and we discuss the direction of our current efforts.

2   Background

In the background section we discuss the hazard analysis techniques and theories that form the basis for the ISHA method [24]. This discussion begins with a brief summary of the Failure Modes and Effects family of hazard analysis techniques [28] and of Leveson's system theoretic accidents models and processes (STAMP) [23]. We continue by summarizing our prior work [30,31] which employs Leveson's STAMP theory to model EMR use in the process of care. We then summarize the main steps of the ISHA method. We follow this with an introduction to an ISHA recommended safety factors taxonomy as it is relevant to the development of functionalized safety requirements. Finally, we introduce the electronic medical document exchange for consult/referral use case, the application context for the hazard analysis presented in our current work.

2.1   FMEA and STAMP

The Failure Modes and Effects Analysis (FMEA) family of hazard analysis methods have their roots in the original process created by the US Department of Defense at the end of the second world war [26]. Since then, a wide range of authors and analysts have applied, extended and adapted the process in different ways. Stamatis [28], identifies a breadth of these variations including: System, Design, Process, Service and Machine FMEA. Yang and El-Haik [33] discuss Software FMEA (SFMEA) while De Rosier [11] discusses health care FMEA (HFMEA). At a high level these analysis techniques consider the mechanisms which lead to system failure and then consider the impact of those failures. The impact is typically assessed in terms of loss/harm events. Another aspect of these methods is that they often include a criticallity analysis step which is used to prioritize the mitigation of identified failure modes. This process variation is identified by the inclusion of the supplemental step in the moniker: failure modes and effects *criticallity* analysis (FMECA). Given our focus on CIT, the ISHA process was particularly influenced by SFMEA and HFMEA.

One shortcoming of the FMEA methods is their weak support for context consideration. This lead us to supplement our analysis technique with concepts derived from a socio-technical theory developed by Leveson [23] called System Theoretic Accidents Models and Processes (STAMP). Leveson developed STAMP in part to address weaknesses of commonly adopted preceding accident analysis techniques such as FMEA [23]. She expresses that context consideration is a central weakness of these methods. She argues that employing event chain analysis when investigating accidents/hazards leads to failures to consider the full breadth of factors which contribute them.

In STAMP, cybernetic systems are modeled as hierarchical control loop webs. The theory incorporates concepts of hierarchical control, feedback, and adaptive systems in a unified framework. Using STAMP, an analyst models a socio-technical system as a set of controllers, displays, controls, sensors, actuators and processes. The controllers connect to the processes they control via input and output links representing control and perception activities. If the process under investigation were controlled directly, then the controller would operate via direct controls and would directly perceive the process state using sensors. On the other hand, if the process were controlled indirectly, the interaction between controls and the controlled process would be mediated by an intermediate controller and an actuator. Information provided to the controller about the controlled process would be provided through displays and would be filtered from the sensors through the intermediary controller. The first scenario is referred to as direct control and perception while the second is referred to as indirect control and synthesized perception. Alternatively, the second scenario is simply referred to as automation. These two models of control are illustrated in Fig. 1

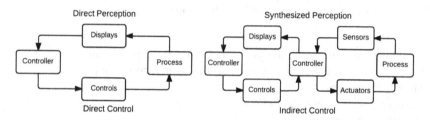

Fig. 1. Leveson's STAMP theory supports the modelling of direct-control/perception (left) and also indirect-control/synthesized-perception (right).

In earlier work, we applied STAMP to generate a general adaptive control model for the use of CIT which is based on an indirect control/synthesized perception paradigm [31]. The model highlights a variety of potential failure modes of these automation systems and provides a system-theoretic lens through which to consider CIT safety issues. This adaptation of Leveson's model is presented in Fig. 2.

2.2   ISHA

The ISHA methodology proceeds through a set of core steps which are similar to those presented in many FMEA derived methodologies. These fundamental phases are enumerated below [24]:

1. Assemble a cross functional and interdisciplinary team
2. Identify the process to analyze

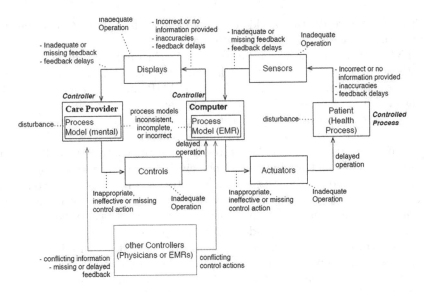

Fig. 2. The figure illustrates a model of EMR use which is based on Leveson's indirect-control/synthesized-perception paradigm. Potential failure modes are highlighted and linked to the model components in which they arise.

3. Scope the system under analysis and formalize scope assumptions
4. Consolidate and revise requirements, and formalize assumptions
5. Model the system
6. Identify failure modes and effects
7. Prioritize failure modes
8. Supplement base requirements with safety-centric requirements
9. Ameliorate, mitigate, and control hazards

In the team assembly phase, an appropriately cross functional team is assembled to analyze the information system under investigation. This team will typically include end users, informations and engineers. Next, the team selects a process for analysis. The selection is informed by available historical accident data or, should such information not be available it is chosen based on a more subjective stratification of processes based on expected risks of loss events. After this, the team scopes the system from a system theoretic perspective while at the same time formalizing the assumptions on which the chosen system scope is based. Subsequently, the requirements of the scoped system must be consolidated from relevant sources including system experts and written documentation, and must also be revised. Next, the system is modeled using a conceptual modeling language to facilitate the subsequent hazard analysis. Once the system has been modeled, failure modes must be identified. The process as expressed in [24] does not prescribe the method by which failure modes are to be identified but rather leaves these decisions to the analysts. In our present work we employ a guide statement driven analysis of each component and of the interactions of components based on Leveson's System Theoretic Process Analysis (STPA) methodology. We also apply the safety factors taxonomy we presented in [24] as a lens with which to identify further failure modes. We illustrate this taxonomy here in Fig. 3. These mechanisms in concert facilitate the systematic generation of a supplemental set of safety-centric requirements for the system.

In the final stages of the process, identified failure modes are prioritized based on the analysts' subjective assessment of their risk levels rather than based on risk priority numbers (RPN) as is prescribed by the FMECA methodology. This divergence is based on the arguments of Shebl [27] who articulated many ways in which RPN based stratification is not mathematically sound. The failure modes are then addressed with amelioration, mitigation and control recommendations in order of priority, and the recommendations are subsequently implemented.

2.3   Safety Factors Taxonomy

The ISHA method requires that we identify/develop a comprehensive list of requirements for the system. While defining the operational goals of actors is relatively straight forward, addressing the qualitative aspects (e.g., safety) is more challenging. In order to facilitate the identification of safety related qualitative attributes of the operational processes, ISHA proposes the application of a guide word strategy as do other methods including Leveson's STAMP derived methodologies [23]. The challenge we faced with this approach is that no comprehensive set of guide words could be identified in the literature. Liu suggested the use of guide words provided in ISO 9126, based in part on the work of McCall [25], but investigation revealed these to be inadequate for this purpose.

This motivated our development of a novel taxonomy of safety [24]. We assembled this taxonomy based on the ISO 9126 [19] standard, the original work of McCall which the standard cited, safety relevant issues identified by Win [32], Alonso-Rios's usability taxonomy [1], and an enrichment phase fueled by our own experience and knowledge. The structure of our taxonomy is grounded in McCall's stratification of software attributes into factors, criteria and metrics. It provides high level factors of safety and then breaks these down into criteria which can qualify the degree to which the system fulfills the factors. Criteria can then be quantified using metrics as proxies to provide evidence of the degree to which the system meets the specified criteria (Fig. 3).

The taxonomy is composed of three core safety factors: integrity, availability and Usability demonstrating clear similarity to the core elements of security - integrity, availability and confidentiality. Integrity is subdivided into three subcategories. Data integrity describes issues with the currency and validity of single datum. Information integrity describes issues with data association. Finally, knowledge integrity describes issues with rules and inferences about the relationship between two or more associated elements of data. Availability addresses the concepts of reliability and fault tolerance. Finally, usability addresses safety related human factors issues and operability which includes functional completeness, interoperability and universality. This final criteria, derived from

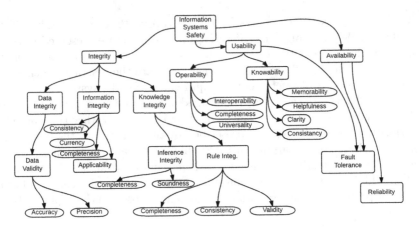

Fig. 3. The safety factors taxonomy recommended by ISHA is based on three core safety factors: usability, integrity and availability. These core factors are further subdivided into subfactors and criteria. The criteria are specific system attributes which are associated with satisfying the core safety factors. The measures used to quantify these criteria are called metrics. Adapted from [24].

Alonso-Rios [1], incorporates the concept of accessibility. The taxonomy is divided into factors in rectangular boxes and criteria in ovals.

2.4   EMR to EMR: The Episodic Document Business Context

The HL7 CDA [12] based E2E specification [16] was recently prescribed for use in British Columbia, Canada. It has been engineered to facilitate the exchange of patient records electronically between a variety of disparate EMR systems and for a constrained set of clinical work flows. The work flows are EMR export for the exchange of full patient sets between EMRs, patient exports which satisfy individual patient transfer needs, episodic documents which fulfill referral and consultation requirements as well as a variety of other care episode driven use cases, and unstructured documents for less structured communications. We focus here on the referral/consult work flow and thus provide an adaptation of the informal model of the episodic document context illustrated in [16] which is specialized to the referral/consult use case to ground the reader (Fig. 4).

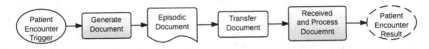

Fig. 4. A first physician encountering a patient identifies the necessity for a consultation. She generates a referral document, and transfers the document to a consulting physician. If the consulting physician accepts the consultation request, he treats the patient. Adapted from [16].

3   Analysis

In the analysis section we will discuss the execution of each phase of the ISHA process. We cover the stages sequentially, but the analysis was iterative. The sequential presentation was chosen to facilitate communication.

3.1   Assembly of the Cross Functional Team

The investigators assembled as a cross functional team to analyze the E2E episodic document business context. Investigators were driven by individual research motivations and contributed to share skills and knowledge across disciplinary boundaries. JW is a licensed software engineer. FMB is a Computer Science PhD candidate. AR is a health informatician. MP is a practicing MD.

3.2   Identify the Process to Analyze

The ISHA method suggests that process selection should ideally be driven by retrospective data and that analysis should focus primarily on work flows that have incurred the most significant incidents. In this case, no past data on E2E was available as the standard is new. We therefore selected the *consult/referral* work flow based on general published evidence that activities which involve transition of care are especially susceptible to medical errors.

3.3   Scope the System Under Analysis

The episodic document business context can be modeled as a webbing of control loops using the STAMP meta-model (controllers, controls, actuators, sensor and displays). A diagram illustrating such a model is shown in Fig. 5. The representation is derived from our STAMP EMR model - Fig. 2. The episodic document model was validated against typical clinical work flow by both MP and by AR.

In this model, both the referring and consulting physician are engaging in both direct and indirect control over their shared patient's health care process. Supplementary to this, each physician is also engaged in direct control of their patient's electronic medical record in their respective local systems, as well as in indirect control of the remote record. This indirect control of the remote patient record is mediated by the episodic document and is filtered by controls, automated and not, which are instituted by the physician who reconciles the incoming documents.

In addition, the interaction between the care providers and their shared patient's health care process is being monitored and controlled by two external classes of controllers: technical process controllers and health care process controllers. The technical controllers include software and hardware vendors as well as technical trainers or other technical supports which may be at work. Though the technical controllers can directly manipulate the health care process by deploying new hardware or software, by modifying training processes, or by

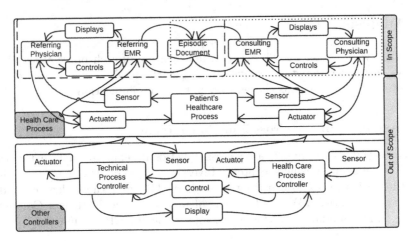

Fig. 5. The episodic document business context is modeled as a webbing of control loops using a meta-model of Leveson's STAMP. The scope of our analysis is primarily limited to clinician interactions with the EMR software as indicated on the right.

providing new technical support systems, they still operate under the auspices of the health care process controllers. This latter class of controllers represents organizations like the governmental health ministry, the local health authority, or even the medical practices' chief information officer. These bodies are involved in the direct control of the health care process as it is their duty to ensure its sufficient functioning. They simultaneously engage in indirect control and synthesized perception of the health care process through their interactions with the technical controllers. For example, they may put constraints on the quality of hardware which can be deployed, or on software functionality.

For our analysis we exclude the technical and health care process controllers. Our focus for this investigation revolves around physician interactions with the EMR software. Consequently, we also provide only limited analysis of clinical practices which do not relate directly to the EMR. What remains in scope are the EMR software, the consulting and referring physicians, these physicians' interactions with the EMR software, the episodic document and finally the document's transmission between the two physicians. These scope boundaries are soft by necessity as hazards related to components inside this scope sometimes depend on components which are outside of it.

3.4   Scope the Requirements Under Analysis

Often, only a subset of relevant requirements and assumptions are clearly and explicitly documented in a form that is accessible for analysis. In our case study of the conceptual architecture of an episodic document exchange system for example, we had to infer use case requirements from a narrative specification [16] and expert advice from AR and MP. We begin by stating the assumptions which we assert. These were motivated by the integrity focus of our analysis and were also chosen to reflect our chosen scope.

As our interest is in integrity, we assert availability and usability which are the other two foundational elements of the ISHA recommended safety factors taxonomy (Fig. 3). The notion of usability we adopt here is derived from the work of Alonso-Rios [1]. As discussed, it incorporates concepts of operability, accessibility, knowability and a variety of other usability aspects. We strengthen these assertions by assuming that care providers are intimately familiar with the software they use, and that they do not make errors of intention. As we have expressed, our focus is on the software primarily, and soft issues that do not relate immediately to the software have been excluded from the scope of our analysis. Lastly, we make further assertions about the capacity and goals of the physicians in question. We assert that physicians can verify and validate the records the system produces. We make this assertion as considerations of issues related to failures in this scenario quickly lead to assessments of the risks in health care more generally. Finally we assert that physicians do not maliciously alter the data in the system. This again is a soft issue, and it could well exist entirely distinct from the software. We summarize our assumptions below.

Assumptions:

1. CIT software devices in our system are highly available.
2. CIT software devices in our system are highly usable [1] in the context of episodic document exchange and care providers are intimately familiar with them.
3. Care providers are able to faithfully verify the integrity of demographic and clinical information which is provided to them by the CIT devices they use.
4. Care providers do not maliciously manipulate clinical content of the CIT.

We now proceed to enumerate the use case level functional requirements which were inferred through analysis of the narrative specification and from discussion. Our analysis remains sufficiently high level at this point that we have not yet leveraged the formal specification of the document structure and contents from the E2E implementation guide [16]. We instead focus on interoperability at the system level. We consider the operability of the subsystems which generate, receive and transmit documents. We also consider both the transmission of documents and the medium of those transmissions. We have not validated that the requirements provided by the narrative specification are the true requirements, but rather accept them as documented fact. We have validated that the requirements we state are those expressed in the narrative specification to the extent that we achieved a consensus amongst the analysis team.

At this stage it is necessary to differentiate further between contexts of care. We differentiate between longitudinal contexts and episodic contexts. Community clinics (e.g., family practices) operate almost exclusively as longitudinal contexts. They monitor a patient over a long period of time, up to and including the patient's full lifespan. Similarly, practices which focus on chronic disease management populate the longitudinal context. On the other hand, emergency

department systems as well as short term consultative practices operate in the
episodic context.

An episodic communication can be initiated by either an episodic system, or
a longitudinal system. For example, a GP may refer a patient to an oncologist
for a suspected lung cancer. The oncologist may determine that the patient
does not in fact have cancer, but determine that they are suffering from chronic
obstructive pulmonary disorder. The oncologist may then refer the patient to a
practice which focuses on longitudinal management of this condition.

With this basis established, we present requirements which were inferred
from the specification [16] and which were then validated through discussion
and consensus amongst the analysts.

Core Requirements:

1. The devices must be capable of storing patient data for subsequent retrieval.
2. The devices must associate patients with their clinical information.
3. The devices must identify sending and receiving care providers.
4. The devices must produce and consume episodic documents.
5. The devices must send and receive episodic documents to referring or consulting care providers.
6. The medium of transmission for the episodic documents must be secure.
7. Longitudinal systems must reconcile episodic document responses.
8. Episodic documents which are exported/imported, sent/received must include all relevant provenance, target, demographic and clinical information.

3.5 Model the System

Based on the identified core requirements, two SysML models of the episodic document business context were developed. The block definition diagram provides a
static perspective of a conceptual system (Fig. 6), while an activity diagram specifies the dynamic behavior (Fig. 7). The two representations are generalizations
of implemented systems which have been inspected by the investigators.

3.6 Identify Failure Modes and Effects

Reproducibly identifying failures and effects is facilitated by the application of
a systematic approach to the process. For this reason, ISHA recommends a two
stage process. In keeping with the failure analysis proposed by Yang and El-Haik
[33], we wish to evaluate the consequence of failing to satisfy functional requirements. To proceed then, we must first consider our core functional requirements;
however, we must also supplement these with any necessary safety requirements.
This presents a challenge however. In order to consider the failure modes and
effects of safety requirements in this same way, we must first functionalize them.

We identify safety requirements by considering the degree to which our system satisfies the safety factors considered in the ISHA recommended safety factors taxonomy (Fig. 3). We formalize and functionalize these requirements and
then consider how these requirements are, or could be, discharged.

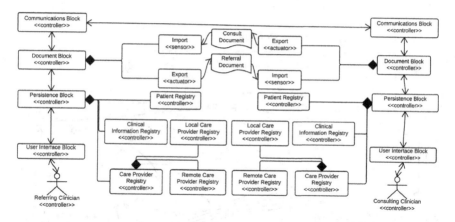

Fig. 6. The episodic document business context involves the interoperation of two disparate EMRs. The systems use communications interfaces to exchange the episodic documents. Each individual conceptual system is comprised of seven core blocks: communication, persistence, document, patient registry, care provider registry, clinical registry, and user interface. The user interfaces are used by the physicians to reconcile medical history with problem updates. The reconciled information is recorded in the registries. These are sourced by the exporter to populate documents. The communications block transmits the documents over the to the intended recipient. The receiving system's importer reconciles the document contents with the local registries. Finally the receiving physician takes action based on the information which is extracted with the user interface.

We then perform a component-wise investigation. We consider the ways that each of the components might lead to a failure to satisfy each requirement. To guide this exercise we rely on Leveson's control analysis guide statements [23]:

1. A control action required for safety is not provided or is not followed
2. An unsafe control action is provided that leads to a hazard
3. A potentially safe control action is provided too late, too early, or out of sequence
4. A safe control action is stopped too soon.

Safety-Centric Requirements. Where safety is concerned we pay special attention to the topic of integrity. This is because the validity, comprehensiveness and correctness of clinical records is fundamental to a clinicians understanding of a patients state of health [17]. Rough requirements were derived by a stepwise consideration of each factor in the ISHA recommended safety taxonomy (Fig. 3) and were subsequently functionalized. A draft of these requirements is listed below. It is acknowledged that at present it is challenging to validate or verify that these requirements are met. This is in part a consequence of the fact that our analysis focuses on the creation, consumption, transmission and exchange of documents and not on their content. It is also in part a consequence of the non-clinical nature of the analysis. Concepts of data association completeness and

Patient Referral

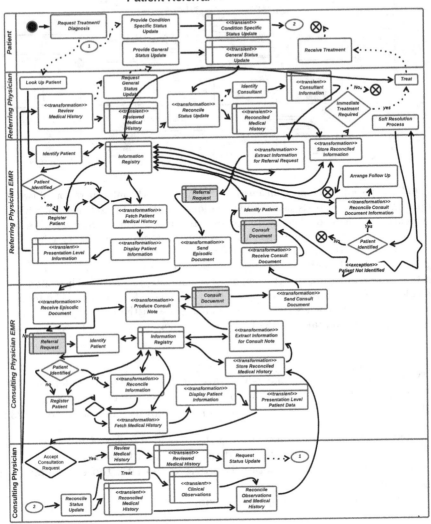

Fig. 7. The episodic document work flow is illustrated using SysML. We simplify our diagram by using bidirectional object flows as a shorthand for pairs of flow relationships in both directions. The process is initiated when a patient encounter triggers the need for the referring physician to request the expertise of a consulting physician. The referring physician uses her EMR to produce and transmit an episodic document. Through this process a number of transformations of the relevant portions of the patient's medical data is performed. Upon the completion of the consultation, the consulting caregiver responds to the referring physician with a consult note similarly producing and subsequently transmitting the document. This stage requires a second, but analogous set of transformations to the patient's now supplemented medical history.

precision are significantly informed by clinical context. The abstract nature of our analysis makes evaluation of these requirements challenging if not impossible. Validation and verification of rule bases, though technical is some senses, is also quite clinical in nature. Our analysis to date is more technical in nature. The issue of latency is also highly context dependent making it challenging to validate. Given clinical context however, a maximum delivery time could be established for certain classes of requests and responses.

Requirements:

1. Documents which are exported by the system must be integral.
    (a) The system must export documents which contain accurate and sufficiently precise data.
    (b) The system must export documents in which the data elements are current, consistent, complete and both completely and consistently associated in a fashion which is relevant to the context of application.
    (c) The system must export documents in which the inferred data that is provided, is inferred from a complete, consistent and valid rule base. The inferences the system uses must also be made soundly and the complete set of relevant inferences must be made and provided.
2. The systems must produce and consume document content without compromising the integrity of that content.
3. Longitudinal systems must reconcile incoming clinical content with existing clinical content without compromising the integrity of that content.
4. Documents must be faithfully delivered to their target recipients.
5. The medium must not compromise the integrity of the document.
    (a) The latency in the combination of the production, transmission and consumption of documents must not compromise their currency.

Model Analysis. We next analyze the degree to which the functional requirements can be discharged to components of the system. We also identify which activities are relevant to their fulfillment in the activity diagram to gain further insight into potential failures. We thus simultaneously consider static and dynamic aspects of the system.

Through analysis we established that the majority of the core requirements can be discharged to both activities and to blocks in our models. The notable exception is requirement 6 - the medium of transmission for the E2E episodic documents must be secure. This is a significant challenge as no single provider will have the capital or inclination to maintain and monitor the communications network over which they share documents with their peers. This aspect of the problem is mitigated in BC as it is prescribed that such communications will be held over a government funded private network. This requires us to consider a technical controller of our system and the support components which they provide in ensuring that the network is secure. It is relevant to our analysis because the medium of transmission influences the integrity of the communicated documents, and thus also impacts the safety of our system.

Where the safety-centric requirements are concerned, the challenges begin to mount. Though a centralized block could handle failure detection, and could even produce signals which could trigger corrective actions, the block could only partially address safety requirements. The handling of failures which arise as a consequence of design process for example, should clearly not be discharged to a block which is produced by that same design system. We propose instead that the many cross cutting ways in which aspects of the safety requirements are discharged need to be identified and explicitly expressed.

Where the specific analysis of our conceptual architecture is concerned, two primary themes arise - communication integrity and content integrity. The communication integrity issues revolve around the completeness of communications. For example, it is hazardous if a referral is not received by a consultant, or if that consultant does not process the referral, or if the consultant does not reply to the referring physician once she has processed the request. We refer to this as the round trip communication problem. The second issue of content integrity has three primary expressions. The first is the identification of patients. Patient missidentification is a well known problem with potentially critical consequences to the patient [29]. The second is problematic record reconciliation. This hazard can present equally catastrophic consequences under the right circumstances. Lastly, there is the case of incorrect or incomplete data. This hazard is interesting in that a large error is better than a small error. If a response from a consultant is empty, it is clear to the recipient that an error has occurred; however, if the response does not include some small number of critical details, things are much worse. Similarly, if the response is not empty, but some of the information is incorrect, the patient is at greater risk. We present a complete reporting of identified hazards at [14].

3.7 Prioritize Failure Modes

The prioritization process taken in our application of the ISHA process emerged organically and was somewhat unexpected. While many FMEA methodologies suggest prioritizing tasks based on risk priority number, we found instead that thoughtful consideration of mechanisms to mitigate effects lead to solutions which would have an impact across much of our system improving the safety of many of its facets simultaneously. In essence, we identified common themes amongst the failure effects and designed solutions which addressed these themes. However, as a consequence of time and space constraints, we were forced to choose one very specific hazard to analyze in detail. We elected to focus on patient missidentification as it is a well known and frequently reported problem [29]. Its selection is also in keeping with the ISHA method - the method prescribes process selection based on historical incident data.

3.8 Ameliorate, Mitigate and Control

A safety focused CIT system should have its safety requirements explicitly discharged to an appropriate set of cross cutting system components. These components should monitor and adjust the safety parameters of the CIT system on the basis of safety margins as quantified using relevant metrics for proxies. Ideally, this feedback loop could run in real time. In current practice, these control loops tend to operate more slowly. They may operate on an episode of care frequency when critical medical errors are made, but when major hazards are identified but not actualized, they are instead typically subject to software development cycle time lines - often measured in months in the EMR domain. Consequently, we take a real time systems control perspective on this problem.

In this work, we specifically address patient missidentification. This hazard was identified from retrospective information [29], and was also identified as a failure mode in our analysis. The failure mode has the potential to lead to two immediate possible effects which have overlapping downstream clinical impact. We refer to the first as a split chart, and the second as a mixed chart.

A split chart occurs when a new record is created for a patient who already has a chart in the system. A mixed chart occurs when a chart not associated with a patient being treated is used to record information about that patient's encounter. Both situations present the hazard that during a subsequent visit, the initial patient will be treated based on incomplete clinical content. With the mixed chart, the problem worsens as this first hazard remains, but the possibility that the patient who's chart was incorrectly modified will now be treated based on incorrect clinical chart content as well. The two problems differ additionally in the nature of the solutions which can address them. Techniques used to address these problems include both prevention and correction.

Where the split chart is concerned, prevention and correction techniques are similar, while with the mixed chart hazard, the nature of correction strategies are likely to differ from detection strategies. When considering the split chart case, similar identities in the system could be presented as match alternatives. Similar strategies could be used to retroactively identify charts for similar recorded identities. These techniques would be primarily syntactic in nature. Where a mixed chart has materialized, an identity based retrospective mechanism cannot be applied without providing details about the identity of the patient who's data was mixed. Thus, if a syntactic approach is taken, additional input beyond the contents of the persistence block must be considered. If this approach is not taken, an analyst could try semantic approaches instead.

The question of amelioration, mitigation and control when it comes to this failure mode requires a refinement of the failure mode definition. Patient missidentification is not a single mode of failure but rather a class of failure modes each of which arise by their own mechanisms. We will address here two concrete manifestations of this mode of failure. In the first we will address a possible failure which might occur in instances where out of province patient identifiers are used. In the second case, we will consider implications of relying on secondary identifiers when they are presented in consult documents which are returned in response to referral requests.

Out of Province Identifiers. One mechanism by which the patient identification failure mode could arise is where an out of province identifier is used to identify the subject of a referral or consult document. The E2E specification prescribes that the subject of a document shall be identified using an id element. The id element has two attributes of significance, a root and an extension. The root identifies the code system and is expressly prescribed to be a universally unique identifier. The extension, though not expressly prescribed to be, is strongly implied to be locally unique to the namespace identified by the root.

Systems are prescribed to use BC Personal Health Number (PHN)'s where possible, but it is permissible to send an identifier from a different code system if a PHN is not available. It is conceivable then, that an extension could be provided in a document identifying a patient using an out of province id. This id may have an analogous format to the BC PHN. If then, the system developers neglected to consider this and hard coded the BC PHN root for all documents, a merged chart could arise. To address such a problem, a multi-field key matching algorithm could be employed in both the document block and the user interface block.

Round Tripping and Secondary Identifiers. A second mechanism by which this failure mode could arise is in shortcut interpretation of values returned from consulting systems. Consider a referring system which provides both a patient's PHN and local identifier. The local system uses a 64-bit integer to represent its identifiers. A referral document is produced and then accepted by a consulting system. The consultant treats the patient and responds. The consulting system meanwhile has stored all the information provided in the referral document. The consulting system however considers all ids to be 32-bit integers. The resulting truncation at storage compromises the identifier. Consider now that the consulting system may respond with a consult document to the referring system who relies on the secondary identifier in consult documents. The document is a response, therefore it may appear fair to assume that if the content remains, the content is unchanged. This could result in a split chart if no patient exists with the truncated local identifier, or a merged chart if such a patient does exist.

To mitigate such a possibility, the referring system could institute a policy by which a check is made to ensure that consult documents are never merged before confirmation is made that a referral has been requested for the matched patient. This is however just another constraint, which could be circumvented through intention or by accident. A significant challenge with safety design is that accidents can arise as a consequence of a factor, or an alignment of factors about which system controllers are ignorant.

4   Conclusions and Current Work

Despite the safety-critical role of HIT, hazard analyses of these systems are sparsely reported. We have presented a hazard analysis of the episodic document context using ISHA, an FMEA/STAMP-based method specifically geared for analyzing hazards in critical information systems. This process produced a number of recommendations for our conceptual system design. A summary of a small number of these hazards was presented. At the moment our hazard analysis is purely based on the E2E standards documentation and generic requirements. The next step will be to consider implementations of E2E functionality of EMR vendor products. This analysis should include consideration of document contents as well as the aspects of document exchange which we considered here. We currently collaborate with a number of EMR vendors in the province which have implemented the E2E standard and we have begun to investigate the safety properties of E2E implementations in two of these systems so far. This work is ongoing.

Another line of research is the further refinement, formalization and tooling of the ISHA method. In our application, the opportunity for reproducibility issues arose in the requirements definition phase in spite of our efforts to employ a systematic requirements consolidation process. The method does not explicitly address differences between design and redesign applications, nor does it provide clear guidance on how to manage functional vs safety requirements. In fact it suggests that analysts avoid making such a distinction; this is challenging in practice. Further, the requirements consolidation and modeling steps in typical software engineering processes are iterative and interlinked. The methodology prescribes that the steps be performed sequentially. Further criticism still could be leveled at the ISHA process in considering the recommended guide word approach to identifying failure modes. Though Leveson's [23] guide words are well informed and valuable, other guidewords like those in the SAE Architecture Analysis and Design Language Error Model Language, could be considered.

We have focused here exclusively on integrity. Different problems and solutions would be identified if integrity were asserted and availability or usability were investigated. Such an exploration could provide additional depth and breadth of understanding of the nature of safety in socio-technical systems which implement CIT.

References

1. Alonso-Ríos, D., Vázquez-García, A., Mosqueira-Rey, E., Moret-Bonillo, V.: Usability: a critical analysis and a taxonomy. Int. J. Hum. Comput. Interact. **26**(1), 53–74 (2009)
2. Ash, J.S., Sittig, D.F., Dykstra, R.H., Guappone, K., Carpenter, J.D., Seshadri, V.: Categorizing the unintended sociotechnical consequences of computerized provider order entry. Int. J. Med. Inform. **76**(Supplement 1), S21–S27 (2007). Information Technology in Health Care: Sociotechnical Approaches ITHC 2004
3. Ash, J.S., Sittig, D.F., Poon, E.G., Guappone, K., Campbell, E., Dykstra, R.H.: The extent and importance of unintended consequences related to computerized provider order entry. J. Am. Med. Inform. Assoc. **14**(4), 415–423 (2007)
4. Bogner, M.S.: Revisiting to ERR is human a decade later. Biomed. Instrument. Technol. **43**(6), 476–478 (2009)
5. Bonnabry, P., Cingria, L., Ackermann, M., Sadeghipour, F., Bigler, L., Mach, N.: Use of a prospective risk analysis method to improve the safety of the cancer chemotherapy process. Int. J. Qual. Health Care **18**(1), 9–16 (2006)

6. Bonnabry, P., Cingria, L., Sadeghipour, F., Ing, H., Fonzo-Christe, C., Pfister, R.E.: Use of a systematic risk analysis method to improve safety in the production of paediatric parenteral nutrition solutions. Qual. Safe. Health Care **14**(2), 93–98 (2005)

7. Bonnabry, P., Despont-Gros, C., Grauser, D., Casez, P., Despond, M., Pugin, D., Rivara-Mangeat, C., Koch, M., Vial, M., Iten, A., et al.: A risk analysis method to evaluate the impact of a computerized provider order entry system on patient safety. J. Am. Med. Inform. Assoc. **15**(4), 453–460 (2008)

8. Borycki, E., Keay, E.: Methods to assess the safety of health information systems. Healthc. Q. **13**, 49–54 (2010)

9. Clancy, C.M.: Ten years after to Err is human. Am. J. Med. Qual. **24**(6), 525–528 (2009)

10. Coiera, E., Aarts, J., Kulikowski, C.: The dangerous decade. J. Am. Med. Inform. Assoc. **19**(1), 2–5 (2012)

11. DeRosier, J., Stalhandske, E., Bagian, J.P., Nudell, T.: Using health care failure mode and effect analysis: the VA national center for patient safety's prospective risk analysis system. Joint Comm. J. Qual. Patient Saf. **28**(5), 248–267 (2002)

12. Dolin, R.H., Alschuler, L., Boyer, S., Beebe, C., Behlen, F.M., Biron, P.V., Shabo, A.: Hl7 clinical document architecture, release 2. J. Am. Med. Inform. Assoc. **13**(1), 30–39 (2006)

13. Dückers, M., Faber, M., Cruijsberg, J., Grol, R., Schoonhoven, L., Wensing, M.: Safety and risk management interventions in hospitals a systematic review of the literature. Med. Care Res. Rev. **66**(6 suppl), 90S–119S (2009)

14. Price, M., Roudsari, A., Mason-Blakley, F., Weber, J.: https://connex.csc.uvic.ca/access/content/group/Simbioses/public/ISHA.xlsx. Accessed Aug 2014

15. Franklin, B.D., Shebl, N.A., Barber, N.: Failure mode and effects analysis: too little for too much? BMJ Qual. Saf. **21**(7), 607–611 (2012)

16. Gordon Point Informatics. E2E business overview. http://www.pito.bc.ca/ete-dtc/. Accessed Aug 2014

17. Holden, R.J.: Cognitive performance-altering effects of electronic medical records: an application of the human factors paradigm for patient safety. Cognit. Technol. Work **13**(1), 11–29 (2011)

18. Horsky, J., Kuperman, G.J., Patel, V.L.: Comprehensive analysis of a medication dosing error related to CPOE. J. Am. Med. Inform. Assoc. **12**(4), 377–382 (2005)

19. ISO. ISO9126. Accessed Mar 2014

20. Kohn, L.: To Err is Human: Building a Safer Health System. National Academy Press, Washington, D.C. (2000)

21. Koppel, R., Metlay, J.P., Cohen, A., Abaluck, B., Localio, A.R., Kimmel, S.E., Strom, B.L.: Role of computerized physician order entry systems in facilitating medication errors. JAMA **293**(10), 1197–1203 (2005)

22. Koppel, R., Wetterneck, T., Telles, J.L., Karsh, B.: Workarounds to barcode medication administration systems: their occurrences, causes, and threats to patient safety. J. Am. Med. Inform. Assoc. **15**(4), 408–423 (2008)

23. Leveson, N.G.: Engineering a Safer World: Systems Thinking Applied to Safety. MIT Press, Cambridge (2012)

24. Mason-Blakley, F., Weber, J., Habibi, R.: Prospective hazard analysis for information systems. In: International Conference on Health Informatics (2014)

25. McCall, J.A.: Quality factors. In: Encyclopedia of Software Engineering (1994)

26. United States Department of Defense. Mil-p-1629 - procedures for performing a failure mode effect and critical analysis

27. Shebl, N.A., Franklin, B.D., Barber, N.: Failure mode and effects analysis outputs: are they valid? BMC Health Serv. Res. **12**(1), 150 (2012)

28. Stamatis, D.H.: Failure Mode and Effect Analysis: FMEA From Theory to Execution. ASQ Press, Milwaukee (2003)
29. Weber-Jahnke, J.H.: A preliminary study of apparent causes and outcomes of reported failures with patient management software. In: Proceedings of the 3rd Workshop on Software Engineering in Health Care, pp. 5–8. ACM (2011)
30. Weber-Jahnke, J.H., Mason-Blakley, F.: The safety of electronic medical record (EMR) systems: what does EMR safety mean and how can we engineer safer systems? ACM SIGHIT Rec. 1(2), 13–22 (2011)
31. Weber-Jahnke, J.H., Mason-Blakley, F.: On the safety of electronic medical records. In: Liu, Z., Wassyng, A. (eds.) FHIES 2011. LNCS, vol. 7151, pp. 177–194. Springer, Heidelberg (2012). doi:10.1007/978-3-642-32355-3_11
32. Win, K.T.: The application of the FMEA risk assessment technique to electronic health record systems (2005)
33. Yang, K., El-Haik, B.: Design for Six Sigma. McGraw-Hill, New York (2003)

Using PVSio-web to Demonstrate Software Issues in Medical User Interfaces

Paolo Masci[1(✉)], Patrick Oladimeji[2], Paul Curzon[1], and Harold Thimbleby[2]

[1] Queen Mary University of London, London, UK
{p.m.masci,p.curzon}@qmul.ac.uk
[2] Swansea University, Swansea, UK
{p.oladimeji,h.thimbleby}@swansea.ac.uk

Abstract. We have used formal methods technology to investigate software and user interface design issues that may induce use error in medical devices. Our approach is based on mathematical models that capture safety concerns related to the use of a device. We analysed nine commercial medical devices from six manufacturers with our approach, and precisely identified 30 design issues. All identified issues can induce use errors that could lead to adverse clinical consequences, such as numbers being incorrectly entered. An issue with formal approaches is in making results accessible to developers, human factors experts and clinicians. In this paper, we use our tool PVSio-web to demonstrate the identified issues: PVSio-web allows us to generate realistic and interactive user interface prototypes from the same mathematical models used for analysis. Users can explore the behaviour of the prototypes by pressing buttons on realistic user interfaces that reproduce the functionality and visual representation of the real devices. Users can examine the device behaviour resulting from any interaction. Key sequences identified from analysis can be used to explore in detail the identified design issues in an accessible way.

1 Introduction

According to the US Food and Drug Administration (FDA) many problems reported in incidents involving medical devices are due to use errors and software defects [2]. For example, in the USA, a recent study conducted by FDA software engineers revealed that software-related recalls had almost doubled in just over five years: 14% in 2005 to nearly 25% in 2011 [16]. While it is usual to attribute software failures to coding errors, the FDA study highlighted that the largest class of problems were actually caused by logic errors in software design.

In the present work, a series of realistic prototypes, based on nine real devices from six different manufacturers, have been developed to demonstrate identified relations between *logic errors in software design* and device behaviours that induce use errors (such as accidentally entering a number 10 times higher than

---

Demo video: "Design issues in medical user interfaces" (https://www.youtube.com/watch?v=T0QmUe0bwL8).

M. Huhn and L. Williams (Eds.): FHIES 2014/SEHC 2014, LNCS 9062, pp. 214–221, 2017.
DOI: 10.1007/978-3-319-63194-3_14

intended) that have potential adverse clinical consequences. These logic errors are due either to incomplete or erroneous system requirements and specification, or design features chosen without considering well-known usability heuristics. All demonstrated issues were validated, and can be reproduced on the real devices using the input key sequences presented in our demonstrative video. Some example issues and input key sequences are illustrated in Sect. 4. The prototypes are run in our tool PVSio-web [12], a graphical environment based on the formal verification system PVS [13]. PVS is a well known industrial-level theorem prover that enables mechanised verification of potentially infinite-state systems. It is based on a typed higher-order logic, and its specification language has many features similar to those of imperative programming languages such as C++.

Formal tools typically produce results in a textual form that is usually inaccessible to engineers, and certainly to human factors specialists or clinicians. In contrast, PVSio-web can be used to examine and realistically animate the results of analysis performed with formal verification tools such as PVS. By using PVSio-web this barrier is eliminated because issues can be explored and demonstrated by interacting with a realistic user interface and watching the device behaviour that results from the interaction. The tool can be used for generating test cases for developed devices, or used at earlier phases of design (e.g., to animate a formally specified functional specification) when the final device is not yet available.

2   Our Formal Methods Approach

The analysis approach involves the following steps (see Fig. 1):

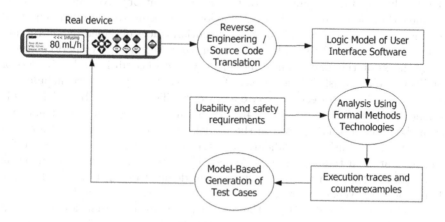

Fig. 1. Our approach for the analysis of user interface software.

– First, a logic model of the device user interface software is developed. It defines how the device supports user actions (e.g., the effect of pressing a button on the user interface), and what feedback (e.g., messages displayed on the screen) is provided to the user in response to user actions or internal device events. These models are obtained from the source code of the device software, or by reverse engineering the device behaviour through systematic interaction with the device.

- Second, the developed model is verified against relevant safety and usability requirements using formal methods technologies — the PVS theorem prover, in this case. Example requirements are: visibility of relevant information about the device state; feedback about what is the current device state and what has been achieved; ability to undo the effect of actions. An illustration of analysed requirements and techniques used to analyse the requirements is in our previous work [3, 6–8]. Within this step, realistic prototypes of the device are automatically generated from the same PVS models using the PVSio-web prototyping environment. The prototypes facilitate model debugging and analysis of conjectures about the device behaviour specified in the model.

- Third, test cases are generated using a semi-automatic approach using graph exploration techniques on the developed model. The aim of these test cases is to validate the model behaviour against the real device, and to check that design issues identified during the analysis apply to the real device and not only to the model. Within this step, prototypes developed with PVSio-web are used to demonstrate the behaviour of the device for the generated input key sequences, and engage with domain and clinical experts to discuss the consequences of identified problematic behaviours.

2.1 Reverse Engineered Models

To perform reverse engineering in a systematic way, we use an iterative approach that involves a direct evaluation of the device behaviour. An initial model is specified that describes the device behaviour according to the documentation provided with the device, and based on execution traces obtained by interacting with the real device. The model is then analysed within PVS to perform basic sanity checks on the model. These include: coverage of conditions; disjointness of conditions; and consistent use of types. To facilitate this analysis, we include pre- and post-conditions for each software feature specified in the PVS model — this is done using predicate subtypes [14], a PVS language mechanism that narrows down the domain of types used in the model. Test cases are generated for each pre- and post-conditions to validate that the behaviour described in the model is consistent with that of the real device. These test cases are given in terms of key presses that can be used with the real device to trigger specific features of the software. Whenever a test case fails on the real device, a discrepancy is identified between the model and the real device. These discrepancies allow us to identify additional conditions that were not taken into account in the model, or actual coding errors in the real device. In the former case, the model is refined, and the process iterated until all tests succeed. In the latter case, the issue is discussed with software engineers, and verified solutions can be identified using the PVS theorem prover.

2.2   Source Code Models

A set of guidelines is used to translate software source code into PVS specifications in a systematic way. The guidelines cover a substantial set of object-oriented language constructs typically used in core software modules. In the following we summarise the guidelines we used for translating C++ source code into PVS specifications.

- Numeric types such as double, float and integer are mimicked in PVS using subtyping [14, 15] — this is needed because the native PVS types are mathematical Reals and Integers.
- Classes and structures are mimicked in PVS using records and datatypes.
- Class variables are emulated in PVS using fields of a user-defined record type, state, that contains a field for each class variable.
- Class functions operating on objects are emulated in PVS as higher-order functions. That is, a PVS function is defined that takes the same types and number of arguments of the corresponding class function; this PVS function returns a new function type that takes a single argument of type state, which emulates the implicit argument of class functions. This modelling approach allows us to maintain the original signature of class functions.
- Conditional statements have identical counterparts in the PVS specification language; iterative statements are translated using recursive functions; sequential statements and local variables used for computation are mocked up using the PVS LET-IN construct that binds expressions to local names.

3   PVSio-web

PVSio-web [12] is our graphical tool for rapid prototyping of user interfaces. The tool can be used at any stage of the development life-cycle for the following purposes: (i) rapid generation of realistic prototypes for exploring design alternatives; (ii) debugging or testing of device models; (iii) demonstration of features of device models; (iv) demonstration of analysis results.

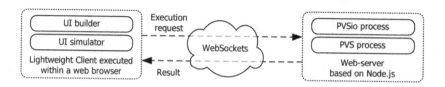

Fig. 2. PVSio-web architecture.

Our tool builds on and extends PVSio [11], the textual simulation environment of PVS. Using PVSio-web, users control PVSio simulations by interacting with buttons and keys of a realistic picture of the device being simulated, and watch the effect of the interactions on the device screen, as in the real device. As illustrated in Fig. 2, the architecture of PVSio-web has two main components: a front-end client, used to interact with the tool; and a back-end server hosting PVS and PVSio. The functionalities of the PVSio-web front-end are now further illustrated.

3.1 Graphical Editor

A snapshot of the PVSio-web graphical editor is in Fig. 3. Using the graphical editor, designers can select a picture of the device being modelled in PVS, and define interactive areas over the picture for identifying input widgets (e.g., buttons, keys) and output widgets (e.g., displays, LEDs). For input widgets, designers can specify which user gestures need to be captured (e.g., clicks), and which PVSio commands need to be invoked for each gesture (e.g., in the picture in Fig. 3, function click_up of the PVS model is executed when the user clicks on the interactive area defined over button ⌃). For output widgets, designers can associate the widget with state variables of the PVS model (e.g., in Fig. 3 a state variable display representing information about the infusion rate is associated to a display area). The PVS model can also be viewed and edited within the graphical editor, using the *PVS editor* bundled with PVSio-web.

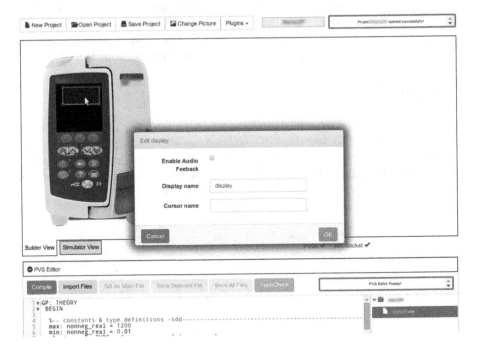

Fig. 3. Snapshot of the graphical editor bundled with PVSio-web. Shaded areas over the picture represent interactive areas for input and output widgets. The form shown upfront allows designers to configure the selected interactive area.

3.2 Simulator

The PVSio-web graphical simulation environment captures user gestures on interactive areas, and renders the current value of state variables during the simulation. Gestures are automatically translated into PVSio commands for invoking the evaluation and execution of functions in the PVS model. These commands are generated on the basis of the current value of state variables in the PVS model, and the association between user gestures and PVSio commands defined using the PVSio-web graphical editor.

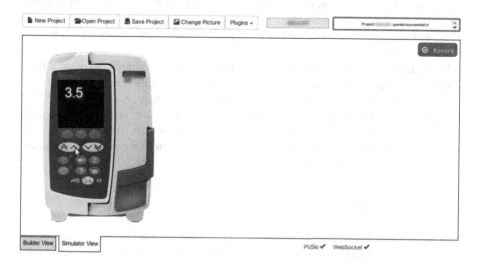

Fig. 4. Example interaction with the PVSio-web simulator: the user clicks on virtual device buttons, and watches feedback on the virtual device display.

A snapshot of the graphical simulation environment during the execution of a simulation is in Fig. 4. It shows an example interaction with the prototype: the user clicks on the virtual device button ⌃, and the effect of this action on the current device state is watched on the virtual device display.

4 Demonstration of Software Design Issues

The developed prototypes demonstrate over 30 software design issues inducing use errors that have potential adverse clinical consequences. The demonstrated device behaviours can be reproduced on commercial medical devices in use in hospitals across the US and UK. Several issues are common in devices from different manufacturers, and across different device types. Here, representative examples of identified issues are presented. The full list of identified issues and an explanation of the consequences of the issues is in our demonstrative video (at https://www.youtube.com/watch?v=T0QmUe0bwL8). A detailed discussion of tools and techniques used to identify these software issues is in [1,3,4,7–9].

- **Decimal point key presses ignored without any warning.** The device registers a key sequence such as ⒈⓪⓪•⒈ as 1,001 (instead of 100.1) without warning. This may cause missing decimal point errors which results in the transcribed number being ten times larger than that intended.
- **Ill-formed values accepted and displayed.** The device shows fractional numbers without a leading zero (e.g., .9 instead of 0.9), or integer numbers with a leading zero (e.g., 09 instead of 9). These cases violate the recommendations issued by the Institute for Safe Medication Practices (ISMP) and may cause numbers to be misread and misinterpreted [5].
- **Entered values ignored without any warning.** If the user fails to confirm the entered value or pauses data entry for a period of time, the device discards the entered value without any warning. This may cause misconfiguration of device parameters.
- **Unintended values rollover.** When the maximum value is overshot with a key press, the value rolls over to the minimum value and vice versa. This may cause misconfiguration of device parameters. Recently, a safety notice [10] involved this design issue. According to the safety notice, there were reported incidents of users accidentally misprogramming an insulin pump to deliver the maximum bolus amount because of this design issue. One of these incidents resulted in severe hypoglycemia.

5 Conclusions

This paper presents the use of formal methods technologies for modelling, simulating and testing safety critical interactive interfaces such as those of commercial infusion devices in use in hospitals. Over 30 software design issues are demonstrated that may create traps for the users that can lead to use error during interactions with the device. Occurrences of these errors can have consequences on patient safety — therefore, these issues should be identified and dealt with.

The presented results were obtained from retrospective analysis of existing device designs. Our analysis tools and techniques, however, can be used at earlier stages of the development process when the software for the real device is not yet implemented. While traditionally there has been poor communication between formal methods experts and human factors experts, our tool and analysis methods take a step towards bridging this gap, as they provide an accessible approach for reasoning about the safety and usability of a product using rapid prototyping techniques and realistic simulations.

Acknowledgements. Paul Jones and Yi Zhang (FDA), Julian Goldman and Dave Arney (Massachusetts General Hospital MD PnP Lab, mdpnp.org), Marc Bloom and staff members of the Washington Adventist Hospital, and Paul Lee (Morriston Hospital, Swansea) helped us to validate our findings. This work is supported by EPSRC as part of CHI+MED (Computer-Human Interaction for Medical Devices [EP/G059063/1]).

References

1. Cauchi, A., Gimblett, A., Thimbleby, H.W., Curzon, P., Masci, P.: Safer 5-key number entry user interfaces using differential formal analysis. In: 26th Annual BCS Interaction Specialist Group Conference on People and Computers (BCS-HCI), pp. 29–38. British Computer Society (2012)
2. Center for Devices and Radiological Health: US Food and Drug Administration. Infusion Pump Improvement Initiative, White Paper (2010)
3. Harrison, M.D., Campos, J.C., Masci, P.: Reusing models and properties in the analysis of similar interactive devices. In: Innovations in Systems and Software Engineering, pp. 1–17 (2013)
4. Harrison, M.D., Masci, P., Campos, J.C., Curzon, P.: Demonstrating that medical devices satisfy user related safety requirements. In: 4th International Symposium on Foundations of Healthcare Information Engineering and Systems (2014)
5. Institute for Safe Medication Practices (ISMP). List of error-prone abbreviations, symbols and dose designations (2006)
6. Masci, P., Ayoub, A., Curzon, P., Harrison, M.D., Lee, I., Thimbleby, H.W.: Verification of interactive software for medical devices: PCA infusion pumps and FDA regulation as an example. In: 5th ACM SIGCHI Symposium on Engineering Interactive Computing Systems (EICS 2013). ACM Digital Library (2013)
7. Masci, P., Rukšėnas, R., Oladimeji, P., Cauchi, A., Gimblett, A., Li, Y., Curzon, P., Thimbleby, H.W.: On formalising interactive number entry on infusion pumps. ECEASST **45** (2011)
8. Masci, P., Rukšėnas, R., Oladimeji P., Cauchi, A., Gimblett, A., Li, Y., Curzon, P., Thimbleby, H.W.: The benefits of formalising design guidelines: a case study on the predictability of drug infusion pumps. In: Innovations in Systems and Software Engineering, pp. 1–21 (2013)
9. Masci, P., Zhang, Y., Jones, P., Curzon, P., Thimbleby, H.: Formal verification of medical device user interfaces using PVS. In: Gnesi, S., Rensink, A. (eds.) FASE 2014. LNCS, vol. 8411, pp. 200–214. Springer, Heidelberg (2014). doi:10.1007/978-3-642-54804-8_14
10. Medtronic. Device safety information: accidental misprogramming of insulin delivery (2014). http://www.medtronicdiabetes.com. Report # 930M12226-011
11. Munoz, C.: Rapid prototyping in PVS. National Institute of Aerospace, Hampton, VA, USA, Technical report NIA, 3 (2003)
12. Oladimeji, P., Masci, P., Curzon, P., Thimbleby, H.W.: PVSio-web: a tool for rapid prototyping device user interfaces in PVS. In: 5th International Workshop on Formal Methods for Interactive Systems (FMIS 2013) (2013). http://pvsioweb.org/
13. Owre, S., Rajan, S., Rushby, J.M., Shankar, N., Srivas, M.: PVS: combining specification, proof checking, and model checking. In: Alur, R., Henzinger, T.A. (eds.) CAV 1996. LNCS, vol. 1102, pp. 411–414. Springer, Heidelberg (1996). doi:10.1007/3-540-61474-5_91
14. Rushby, J., Owre, S., Shankar, N.: Subtypes for specifications: predicate subtyping in PVS. IEEE Trans. Softw. Eng. **24**(9), 709–720 (1998)
15. Shankar, N., Owre, S.: Principles and pragmatics of subtyping in PVS. In: Bert, D., Choppy, C., Mosses, P.D. (eds.) WADT 1999. LNCS, vol. 1827, pp. 37–52. Springer, Heidelberg (2000). doi:10.1007/978-3-540-44616-3_3
16. Simone, L.K.: Software-related recalls: an analysis of records. Biomed. Instrum. Technol. **47**(6), 514–522 (2013). doi:10.2345/0899-8205-47.6.514

A Tool for Analyzing Clinical Datasets as *Blackbox*

Nafees Qamar[1]([✉]), Yilong Yang[2], Andras Nadas[1],
Zhiming Liu[3], and Janos Sztipanovits[1]

[1] Institute for Software Integrated Systems, Vanderbilt University, Nashville, USA
{nqamar,nadand,sztipaj}@isis.vanderbilt.edu
[2] University of Macao, Zhuhai, China
yylonly@acm.org
[3] Birmingham City University, Birmingham, UK
zhiming.liu@bcu.ac.uk

Abstract. We present a technique for the automatic identification of clinically-relevant patterns in medical datasets. To preserve patient privacy, we propose and implement the idea of treating medical dataset as a *black box* for both internal and external users of data. The proposed approach directly handles clinical data queries on a given medical dataset, unlike the conventional approach of relying on the data *de-identification* process. Our integrated toolkit combines software engineering technologies such as Java EE and RESTful web services, which allows exchanging medical data in an unidentifiable XML format and restricts users to computed information. Existing techniques could make it possible for an adversary to succeed in data *re-identification* attempts by applying advanced computational techniques; therefore, we disallow the use of retrospective processing of data. We validate our approach on an endoscopic reporting application based on openEHR and MST standards. The implemented prototype system can be used to query datasets by clinical researchers, governmental or non-governmental organizations in monitoring health care services to improve quality of care.

1 Introduction

Patients' Electronic Health Records (EHRs) are stored, processed, and transmitted across several healthcare platforms and among clinical researchers for on-line diagnostic services and other clinical research. This data dissemination serves as a basis for prevention and diagnosis of a disease and other secondary purposes such as health system planning, public health surveillance, and generation of anonymized data for testing. However, exchanging data across organizations is a non-trivial task because of the embodied potential for privacy intrusion. Medical organizations tend to have confidential agreements with patients, which strictly forbid them to disclose any identifiable information of the patients. Health Insurance Portability and Accountability Act (HIPAA) explicitly states the confidentiality protection on health information that any sharable EHRs system must

M. Huhn and L. Williams (Eds.): FHIES 2014/SEHC 2014, LNCS 9062, pp. 222–238, 2017.
DOI: 10.1007/978-3-319-63194-3_15

legally comply with. To abide by these strict regulations, data custodians generally use de-identification[1] techniques [11, 20, 21] so that any identifiable information on patient's EHR can be suppressed or generalized.

However, in reality, research [19] indicates that 87% of the population of U.S. can be distinguished by sex, date of birth and zip code. We can define quasi-identifiers as the background information about one or more people in the dataset. If an adversary has knowledge of these quasi-identifiers, it can possibly recognize an individual and take advantage of his clinical data. On the other hand, we can find out most of these quasi-identifiers have statistical meanings in clinical research. There exists a paradox between reducing the likelihood of disclosure risk and retaining the data quality. For instance, if information related to patients' residence was excluded from the EHR, it would disable related clinical partners to catch the spread of a disease. Thus, strictly filtered data may lead to failure in operations. Conversely, releasing data including patients' entire information including residence, sex and date of birth would bring a higher disclosure risk.

In this paper we address the emerging problem of de-identification techniques, namely, the problem of offering de-identified dataset for a secondary purpose that makes it possible for a prospective user to perform retrospective processing of medical data endangering patient privacy. Figure 1 overviews the proposed technique, and the standard data request process. Our approach differs from the traditional techniques in the sense that it employs software engineering principles to isolate and develop key requirements of data custodians and requesters. We apply Service-Oriented Architecture (SOA) that provides an effective solution for connecting business functions across the web—both between and within enterprises [8].

We also present a prototype of our evolving toolset, implemented using web services to handle data queries. The results are retrieved in an XML data format that excludes all personal information of patients. The basic model used here follows the principles of RESTful web services by combining three elements: a *URLs repository* for identifying resources uniquely corresponding to clinical data queries, *service consumers* requesting data, and *service producers* as custodians of clinical data. The idea of combining web services with SQL queries is although not new, but it tends to provide a technological approach to avoid medical data re-identification risks. The implemented toolkit uses Java EE that offers an easy way to develop applications using EJBs. Needless to mention that Java EE is widespread and is largely used by community.

Our proof-of-concept implementation uses GastrOS, an openEHR [7] database[2] describing an endoscopic application. The underlying technique provides the ability to construct or use stored queries on a clinical dataset. Employing this clinical toy data warehouse of the GastrOS prototype is a useful way to demon-

---

[1] De-identification process is defined as a technology to delete or remove the identifiable information such as name, and SSN from the released information, and suppress or generalize quasi-identifiers, such as zip code date of birth, to ensure that medical data is not re-identifiable (the reverse process of de-identification.).

[2] http://gastros.codeplex.com.

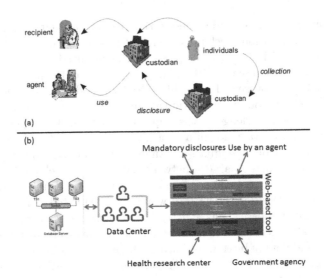

Fig. 1. (a) shows a traditional lifecycle of medical datasets. Custodians can be hospitals, agents may be entities working on their behalf, and recipients are individuals, or organizations such as a pharmaceutical company [5]; (b) depicts the proposed approach that links external entities to data centers using a web interface. The approach excludes all direct data accesses on a dataset.

strate queries on medical data for secondary use. The proposed technique avoids compromising patients' personal information without utilizing de-identification framework tools. For instance, the following query can be posed to GastrOS database using our toolkit:

- Find the number of patients who are still susceptible to developing a Hepatitis B infection even after full compliance to the Hepatitis B vaccination schedule–i.e. the baseline and second detection dates for the HBsAg and Anti-HBs tests both show negative results.

The set of clinical data queries described in the paper have been crafted with the help of clinical researchers at Vanderbilt University. Supporting such complex queries required developing a set of tools, to which this paper provides the first attempt. In contrast to recent developments on big data, this paper does not focus on the management challenges of medical dataset repositories, but rather focuses on software engineering solutions to deal with the challenges of querying medical data endangering patient privacy. Our approach mainly contributes to the development of privacy preserving techniques on patient data by treating datasets as *blackboxes*. In this way, disclosure risks associated with patient data are minimized. One of the key constraints before accomplishing this goal requires keeping the *computability* with data custodians. Relocating datasets is not only unsafe but leads to data re-identification attempts. To ensure that legitimate users access and execute clinical data queries, we implement an authentication and authorization mechanism using role-based access control (RBAC). RBAC offers a flexible architecture that manages users from different organizations by assigning roles and their corresponding permissions.

The paper proceed as follows: Sect. 2 describes the related work; Sect. 3 states an application example; Sect. 4 presents the technical details of our approach; Sect. 5 overviews the clinical data queries corresponding to the GastrOS dataset; Sect. 6 discusses the authentication and authorization mechanism connecting users to clinical datasets; Sect. 7 summarizes the work and details some future research directions.

2   Related Work

In contrast to some of the existing techniques [2,10,12,13,15], our approach relies on advanced software engineering principles and technologies for analyzing clinical datasets. For example, caGrid 1.0 [12] (now caGrid 2.0), released in 2006, is an approach that discusses a complex technical infrastructure for biomedical research through an interconnected network. It aims provide support for discovery, characterization, integrated access, and management of diverse and disparate collections of information sources, analysis methods, and applications in biomedical research. caGrid 1.0 has been initially designed only for cancer research. caGrid combines Grid computing technologies and the Web Services Resource Framework (WSRF) standards to provide a set of core services, toolkits for the development and deployment of new community provided services, and APIs for building client applications. However, caGrid does not focus on an explicit query mechanism to infer details from medical datasets, as the one proposed here. Similar work in [2] discusses a combined interpretation of biological data from various sources. This work, however, considers the problem of continuous updates of both the structure and content of a database and proposes the novel database SYSTOMONAS for SYSTems biology of pseudOMONAS. Interestingly, this technique combines a data warehouse concept with web services. The data warehouse is supported by traditional ETL (extract, transform, and load) processes and is available at http://www.systomonas.de.

De-identification techniques for medical data have been studied and developed by statisticians dealing with integrity and confidentiality issues of statistical data. The major techniques used for data de-identification are (i) CAT (Cornell Anonymization Kit) [21], (ii) μ-Argus [11], and (iii) sdcMicro [20]. CAT anonymizes data using generalization, which is proposed [3] as a method that specifically replaces values of quasi-identifiers into value ranges. μ-Argus is an acronym for Anti-Re-identification General Utility System and is based on a view of safe and unsafe microdata that is used at Statistics Netherlands, which means the rules it applies to protect data comes from practice rather than the precise form of rules. Developed by Statistics Austria, sdcMicro is an extensive system for statistical computing. Like μ-Argus, this tool implements several anonymization methods considering different types of variables. We have reported [9] a comparison on the efficacy of these numerical methods that are used to anonymize quasi-identifiers in order to avoid disclosing individual's sensitive information. The Privacy Analytics Risk Assessment Tool (PARAT)[3] is the only commercial product available so far for de-identifying medical data. Our quantitative analysis [9] of de-identification tools shows that de-identifying data provides no guarantee of anonymity [18]. A study [1] also shows that organizations using data de-identification are vulnerable to re-identification at different rates.

Another approach [10] describes a special query tool developed for the Indianapolis/Regenstrief Shared Pathology Informatics Network (SPIN) and integrated into the Indiana Network for Patient care (INPC). This tool allows retrieving de-identified data sets using complex logic and auto-coded final diagnoses, and it supports multiple types of statistical analyses. However, much of the technical details have not been published; for example, the use of complex logic. This and other similar efforts [14] are mostly database-centric. A slightly similar work to this paper has been developed at Massachusetts General Hospital (QPID Inc.,[4]), offering solutions at a commercial level, but no prototype is available to experiment with. A Web-based approach for enriching the capabilities of the data-querying system is also developed [13] that considers three important aspects including the interface design used for query formulation, the representation of query results, and the models employed for formulating query criteria. The notion of differential privacy [4] aims to provide means to maximize the accuracy of queries from statistical databases while minimizing the chances of identifying its records.

Our analysis shows that the effort to secure medical datasets is mainly two-faceted: (1) most research endeavors have explored the design and development of de-identification tools, and, (2) some work, mostly led by medical doctors, has tried to address the construction of clinical queries, but they do not provide technical details on the construction of their toolsets. Our approach that treats medical datasets as blackboxes mainly considers the automation of services expected from a data custodian in order to minimize data disclosure risks and making clinical datasets easily accessible for internal and external users.

3   GastrOS: An Example Application

GastrOS[5], an openEHR database describing an endoscopic application, is used as a case-study of electronic medical data. This application formed part of the research done at University of Auckland by Koray Atlag in 2010 that investigated software maintainability and interoperability. For this, the domain knowledge model of Archetypes and Templates of openEHR has driven the generation of its graphical user interface. Moreover, the data content depicting the employed terminology, record structure and semantics were based on the Minimal Standard

---

[3] http://www.privacyanalytics.ca/software/.

[4] http://www.qpidhealth.com.

[5] http://gastros.codeplex.com.

Terminology for Digestive Endoscopy (MST) specified by the World Organization of Digestive Endoscopy (OMED) as its official standard.

Employing the clinical toy data warehouse of the GastrOS prototype is a useful way to demonstrate clinical research based queries on medical data for secondary use without compromising patients' personal information by using the approach proposed here. The queries shown here focus on endoscopic findings that provide valuable anonymized information to clinicians. The implemented queries are to be mainly used by medical practitioners and health decision-makers alike to help them in their clinical management of patients at the point-of-care and in formulating appropriate health policies, respectively. For example, the following queries are obtained through brainstorming with medical doctors to illustrate our approach.

- Total number of dialysis endoscopic examination from January 1, 2010 to December 31, 2010.
- Top 5 diagnoses for those patients who received endoscopic examination and the number of cases for each diagnosis from January 1, 2010 to December 31, 2010.
- Age profile of endoscopic patients from January 1, 2010 to December 31, 2010? i.e. number of dialysis patients belonging to each of the age bracket [below 18; 18 to below 40; 40 to below 60; 60 and above.
- Number of patients who are still susceptible to developing a Hepatitis B infection even after full compliance to the Hepatitis B vaccination schedule?–i.e., the baseline and second detection dates for the HBsAg and Anti-HBs tests both show negative results.

The queries given above are only a subset of original queries. The database structure of GastrOS application is described below.

3.1 GastrOS Data Structure

Figure 2 describes the data structure of the GastrOS database. GastrOS database contains the following tables: the clinicaldetection (doctor detection records), patient (patient information), and examination (examination records) tables are stored in the database.

The patient table has two relations: one patient may have more than one clinical detection record or examination record by doctor(s), so the patient id is added as a foreign key in tables ClinicalDection and Examination. GastrOS is a toy database example with insufficient amount of data available. The original database contains less than 20 rows in each table that makes is not useful for our SQL queries. Therefore, we automatically generated virtual data of 10,000 entries (note that any real data on patients also cannot be published.). An example of the generated data is given in Fig. 3. Table 1 provides the up-to-date information on the number of entries in each column of the GastrOS database.

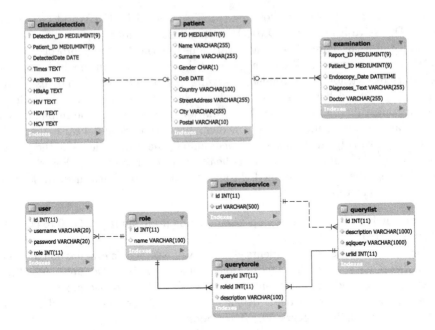

Fig. 2. E-R diagram

Table 1. Generated data in tables

Table	Row	Size
ClinicalDetection	6,393	432 KB
Examination	2,020	272 KB
Patient	1,881	224 KB
Sum	10,294	928 KB

PID	Name	Surname	Gender	DoB	Country	StreetAddress	City	Postal
10000	Adena	Reeves	F	1962-08-28	Montenegro	P.O. Box 936, 9290 Aptent Ave	Morkhoven	71344
10001	Buffy	Warner	M	2009-05-25	Guinea-Bissau	P.O. Box 624, 5536 Nunc St.	Graz	68114-186
10002	Kaye	Green	F	1994-07-23	Norway	P.O. Box 650, 1264 Tellus. St.	Bojano	T04 3WO
10003	Keiko	Gonzalez	M	1973-12-27	Iraq	1889 Magna. Street	Chelsea	8064
10004	Kylynn	Carver	F	1974-01-22	Tanzania	Ap #357-247 Per Rd.	Oberhausen	53534
10005	Daquan	Sosa	F	1961-12-28	Holy See (Vatican City State)	Ap #727-5534 Mauris, Avenue	Eberswalde-Finow	5690ER
10006	Rebekah	Navarro	F	1974-02-01	Saudi Arabia	P.O. Box 698, 3686 Dui. Avenue	Wolvertem	2976
10007	Zane	Benson	M	2002-10-19	Mauritania	Ap #852-3480 Ornare Ave	Dufftown	1137
10008	Jennifer	Petty	F	1985-08-31	Isle of Man	598-2436 Sit Rd.	Bathurst	71612

Fig. 3. Data generated of patient table

4   The Proposed Technique

The proposed approach implements a three-tier application and is devoid of releasing medical datasets, as opposed to traditional techniques. The major purpose and characteristic of the technique extends relatively new software technologies for supporting clinical data queries. In order to support clinical queries under consideration, we develop an integrated application using SOA and Java EE (Enterprise Edition), to extract data from GastrOS database. There are a plenty of other commercial containers such as JBOSS (Redhat), Websphere (IBM), Weblogic and Glassfish (Oracle), which could be used for our purpose. However, our prototype tool combines Java EE based on JSF Primeface, EJB, and Java Persistence Architecture API (JPA). JPA is a Java specification for accessing, persisting, and managing data between Java objects/classes and a relational database.

REST architecture, underlying RESTful web services, treats everything as a resource and is identified by an URI. Resources are handled using POST, GET, PUT, DELETE operations that are identical to Create, Read, Update and Delete (CRUD) operations. Note that in our toolkit it is suffice to implement Read operations for handling the described queries. Every request from a client is handled independently, and it must contain all the required information to interpret the request.

5   Implementing Clinical Queries Using SOA

Web-based authorization and authentication is enforced using role-based access control, before allowing any queries to be accessible by external entities. For instance, the first two queries are shown in Fig. 4. They are linked to Organization A, that shows a limited access varying according to the enabled permissions

id	Description	SQL Query	Service URL	Running Along	Running with Ajax
2	Top 5 diagnoses for those patients who received endoscopic examination and the number of cases for each diagnosis from January 1, 2010 to December 31, 2010.	SELECT Diagnoses_Text, COUNT(Diagnoses_Text) AS Num FROM Examination GROUP BY Diagnoses_Text HAVING COUNT(Diagnoses_Text) >0 LIMIT 5	rws/querytwo	RunNoA	▸ RunA
3	Age profile of endoscopic patients from January 1, 2010 to December 31, 2010 – i.e. Number of dialysis patients belonging to each of the age bracket [below 18; 18 to below 40; 40 to below 60; 60 and above]	SELECT * FROM (SELECT DISTINCT COUNT(PID) AS NumBelow18 FROM Patient, Examination WHERE Patient.PID = Examination.Patient_ID AND YEAR(CURRENT_DATE()) - YEAR(DoB) <18) AS NumBelow18, (SELECT DISTINCT COUNT(PID) AS Num18to40 FROM Patient, Examination WHERE Patient.PID = Examination.Patient_ID AND YEAR(CURRENT_DATE()) - YEAR(DoB) BETWEEN 18 AND 40) AS Num18to40, (SELECT DISTINCT COUNT(PID) AS Num40to60 FROM Patient, Examination WHERE Patient.PID = Examination.Patient_ID AND YEAR(CURRENT_DATE()) - YEAR(DoB) BETWEEN 40 AND 60) AS Num40to60, (SELECT DISTINCT COUNT(PID) AS NumAbove60 FROM Patient, Examination WHERE Patient.PID = Examination.Patient_ID AND YEAR(CURRENT_DATE()) - YEAR(DoB) >60) AS NumAbove60	rws/querythree	RunNoA	▸ RunA

EHR System - Version 2.0

Fig. 4. Query list for role of organization A

by a security administrator. Listing 1.1 shows the result of applied query. SQL queries, exception results, and running time are presented in columns 1, 2, and 3, respectively.

Listing 1.1. Generated XML data

```xml
<?xml version="1.0" encoding="utf-8"?>
<dataset>
 <item>
  <element>
    Diagnoses_Text Colon: Primary malignant tumor,
    Quiescent Crohn's disease
  </element>
  <element>421</element>
 </item>
 <item>
  <element>
    Diagnoses_Text Esophagus: Normal, Ectopic gastric mucosa
  </element>
  <element>394</element>
 </item>
 <item>
  <element>Esophagus: Reflux esophagitis</element>
  <element>414</element>
 </item>
 <item>
  <element>Esophagus: Varices certain</element>
  <element>406</element>
 </item>
 <item>
  <element>Esophagus:Barrett's esophagus</element>
  <element>365</element>
 </item>
</dataset>
```

Note that XML-based format is devoid of platform and programming language dependencies. Using this Web-based approach a diverse set of queries can be supported to query clinical data repositories. For the RESTful-based web services before executing a query, it should have a URL stored in database, that is the table urlforwebservice.

A code snippet is given in Listing 1.2 that reveals how the SQL queries are constructed. Note that all the data saved in a program are objects; nonetheless, our database has actually been represented in the form of relational tables. For this, it needs to implement some ORM (Object-Relational Mapping) techniques. In our prototype implementation we have used JPA (Java Persistence API), because it comes with Java EE technique framework and can be run in either native SQL, or in an object form to allow data manipulation. For instance, we show a *service* code snippet 1.2. @Path show the URL address for this web service, @GET is the method of Restful-based web service, that can be used for other reasons such as @UPDATE @DELETE @POST. Upon invoking a web service using URL in browser or a session bean, the SQL can be executed and return result by query method which invokes the entity manager of JPA.

Listing 1.2. Java code of web service

```
\\For the code of Restful-based web service.
@Path("queryone")
public class QueryOne {
    @Context
    private UriInfo context;
    @EJB
    QueryBean bean;
    @GET
    @Produces("application/xml")
    public String getHtml() {
        // TODO return proper representation object
        String sql = "select Country, COUNT(Report_ID ) AS" +
            "TotalNum" +
            "FROM examination, patient" +
            "WHERE examination.Patient_ID =" +
            "patient.PID" +
            "AND Endoscopy_Date" +
            "BETWEEN \'2010-1-1\'" +
            "AND \'2010-12-30\'" +
            "GROUP BY Country " +
            "Order By TotalNum desc";
        String f = bean.query(sql);
        return f;
    }
}
\\For the method query:
public String query(String sql)
{
    String result = "";
    Query query = emf.createEntityManager().
        createNativeQuery(sql);
    @SuppressWarnings("unchecked")
    List<Object[]> list = query.getResultList();
        ......
}
```

XML data retrieved for a couple of queries are shown in Listings 1.1 and 1.3. The corresponding queries are given below, respectively.

- Top 5 diagnoses for those patients who received dialysis treatment and the number of cases for each diagnosis from January 1, 2010 to December 31, 2010.
- Number of patients for each gender who are still susceptible to developing a Hepatitis B infection even after full compliance to the Hepatitis B vaccination

schedule – i.e. The baseline and second detection dates for the HBsAg and Anti-HBs tests both show negative results.

Listing 1.3. Generated XML data

```
<dataset>
<item>
<element>F</element>
<element>184</element>
</item>
<item>
<element>M</element>
<element>192</element>
</item>
</dataset>
```

5.1   Enabling Dynamic Clinical Queries

The construction and execution of clinical queries on a given dataset are implemented through a web-interface of the tool. The interface allows a user to dynamically construct a clinical query on a dataset. Thus, it adds a greater flexibility to the query mechanism in developing user-oriented analysis of a dataset. For instance, Fig. 5 demonstrates how to execute a query such as "total number of dialysis endoscopic examination of a country starting and ending on a particular date, respectively.", followed by the output in Fig. 6.

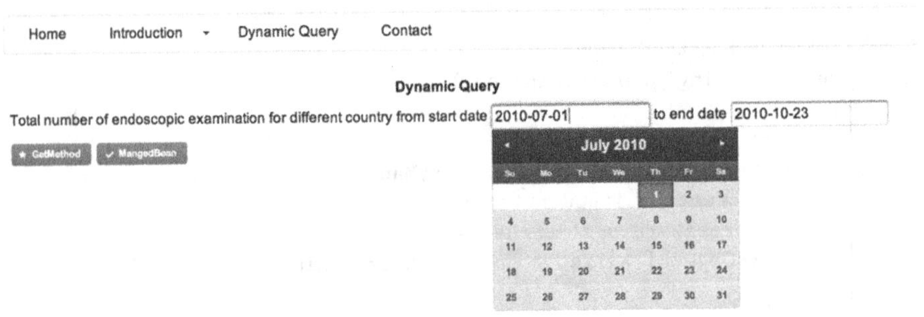

Fig. 5. Interface for executing runtime clinical queries

These queries show that all specific details on patients are avoided when executing a query, which also means that it disables all direct accesses to patient records. It is actually realized by providing a more aggregated form of data on patients instead of conventional techniques that provide medial datasets to infer such details. Note that the toolkit does not allow any query that provides specific

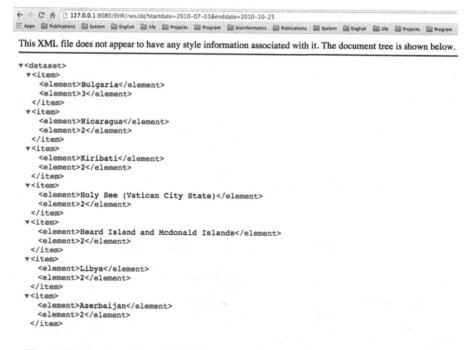

← → C ⌂ 🗋 127.0.0.1:8080/EHR/rws/dq?startdate=2010-07-01&enddate=2010-10-23

⠿ Apps 📁 Publications 📁 System 📁 English 📁 life 📁 Projects 📁 Program 📁 bioinformatics 📁 Publications 📁 System 📁 English 📁 life 📁 Projects 📁 Program

This XML file does not appear to have any style information associated with it. The document tree is shown below.

```
▼<dataset>
  ▼<item>
    <element>Bulgaria</element>
    <element>3</element>
  </item>
  ▼<item>
    <element>Nicaragua</element>
    <element>2</element>
  </item>
  ▼<item>
    <element>Kiribati</element>
    <element>2</element>
  </item>
  ▼<item>
    <element>Holy See (Vatican City State)</element>
    <element>2</element>
  </item>
  ▼<item>
    <element>Heard Island and Mcdonald Islands</element>
    <element>2</element>
  </item>
  ▼<item>
    <element>Libya</element>
    <element>2</element>
  </item>
  ▼<item>
    <element>Azerbaijan</element>
    <element>2</element>
  </item>
```

Fig. 6. The retrieved data in XML format corresponding to the query in Fig. 5

information on patients, such as "Provide details of all patients with a certain age". These queries are directly irrelevant to researchers since they are mainly interested in collective analysis on a dataset. The idea of combining web services with SQL queries is although not new, but it tends to provide a technological solution to a technological problem avoiding medical data re-identification risks. The rationale Using Java EE stems from the fact that it provides an easy way to develop applications, for example, EJB are convenient to use by adding only one annotation. Java EE is also widespread being largely used both in academia and industry.

6   Authentication and Authorization Process

Our prototype system implements role-based access control [6], effectively employed in our previous works [16,17]. For example, for a medical dataset, operations might include insert, delete, append, and update. The data model of RBAC is based on five data types: users, roles, objects, permissions and executable operations by users on objects.

A sixth data type, session, is used to associate roles temporarily to users. A role is considered a permanent position in an organization whereas a given user can be switched with another user for that role. Thus, rights are offered to roles instead of users. Roles are assigned to permissions that can later be

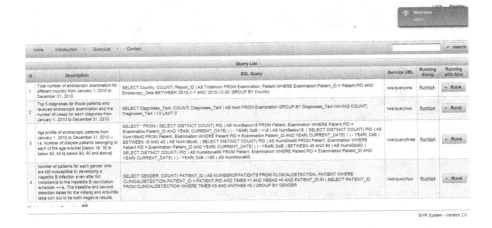

Fig. 7. Query list for role of administrator

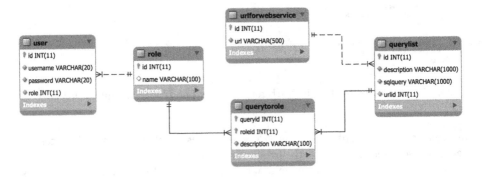

Fig. 8. E-R diagram

exercised by users playing these roles. Modeled objects in RBAC are potential resources to protect. Operations are viewed as application-specific user functions. For example, Fig. 7 shows a list of queries provided to an administrator role.

To maintain a set of permissions on GastrOS database, we use the constructs from RBAC maintain, and enlist entries in corresponding tables users, roles, textsfquerytoroles, querylist, and urlforwebservice. The database tables include user, role, querylist, querytorole, and urlwebservice. We create a user account in user table with the assigned role. Here, all the roles are defined in role table. Users privileges and a list of queries are defined in tables querytorole and querylist, respectively. URLs are stored in the urlwebservice table. For example, logging in as administrator provides five SQL queries shown in Fig. 7, whereas logging in as organization A allows a restricted set of SQL queries as given in Fig. 4. Security management is supervised by an administrator who can do deletion, addition of roles as required. Using RBAC allows users to take multiple roles, for example, the user X could act as researcher that belongs to organization A, but can be assigned another role from the set of roles. Similarly, a permission can be associated to many roles depending on the RBAC policy. The multi-to-multi relation between roles and queries that is given in the querytorole table (Fig. 8).

6.1   Avoiding SQL Injections and Sensitive Information Release

Web application security vulnerabilities occur in cases when an attacker or a authorized user tries to submit and execute a database SQL command on a web application, and thus, a back-end database is exposed to an adversary. These SQL injections can be avoided if queries are validated and filtered before their execution, and are checked against input data or any encoding made by a user. To prevent similar security issue in our web application we first authenticate the user input against a set of defined rules given below:

$$BlockList = \{name, age, address, zipcode\}$$
$$Anti\text{-}injectionList = \{','','', etc.\}$$

Note that the special characters given in a block list helps to avoid SQL injections. The set BlockList disables all possible access to attributes in a table such as name, age, address, and zip code to keep the fetched data completely anonymized. Set members in injectionList filters out three possible vulnerable inputs, i.e., ,, etc. so that any similar attempts could be restricted. Here are the filters that check inputs against BlockList, injectionList. Before running a web service, these two atomic services are always invoked to avoid identifying the actual patients and SQL injections.

– Service one: Checks input string for characters in BlockList.

```
bool CheckDeIdentification(String s)
{
    Check Input string s,
    if it contain character in BlockList,
    return false. Otherwise true.
}
```

– Service two: Checks input string for characters in Anti-injectionList.

```
bool CheckInjection(String s)
{
    Check Input string s,
    if it contain character in Anti-injectionList,
    return false. Otherwise true.
}
```

7   Conclusions and Future Perspectives

We presented a technique for automatic identification of clinically-relevant patterns in medical data. The main contribution of this paper is in defining and presenting an alternative approach to the data de-identification techniques commonly employed for anonymizing clinical datasets. Our technique treats datasets as *blackboxes* and allows data custodians to handle clinical data queries directly. Relocating a dataset not only endangers anonymity of patients, it allows adversaries to apply advanced computational methods for retrospective processing of data. As clinical data is frequently updated, our approach enables data custodians to provide up-to-date resources to their users. We integrate RESTful web services and Java EE with a backend clinical database exchanging anonymous XML data, enabling them to be language and technology independent. Java EE, due to equipped with EJBs, is easy to use for developing applications.

In circumstances related to sharing of patients' data, complex administrative regulations are placed at different levels of management that sometimes unnecessarily complicate the data acquisition process. Providing a tool support for linking data custodians and data requesters using software engineering techniques could pave the way to query clinical datasets more transparently and systematically.

The work provided an initial attempt to build toolset for anonymously analyzing clinical datasets. Our future work includes expanding the approach to more complex databases and supporting an enriched interface for analyzing bigger data repositories. We are currently dealing with the challenge of replacing de-identification techniques in use for de-identifying specific attributes in a database table (e.g. patient ids), for example, a doctor needing to find patients who had an increase of systolic blood pressure within a specific period, or patients with steady states of diastolic blood pressure for more than a week. Our ongoing work considers incorporating such queries into our evolving toolset. We plan to implement ETL processes such as in data warehouses to support clinical data analyses on large-scale integrated databases.

Acknowledgments. The work presented in this paper was funded through National Science Foundation (NSF) TRUST (The Team for Research in Ubiquitous Secure Technology) Science and Technology Center Grant Number CCF-0424422. Its contents are solely the responsibility of the authors and do not necessarily represent the official views of the NSF. This work has been partly supported by the project SAFEHR of Macao Science and Technology Development Fund (MSTDF) under grant 018/2011/AI.

References

1. Benitez, K., Malin, B.: Evaluating re-identification risks with respect to the hipaa privacy rule. JAMIA **17**(2), 169–177 (2010)
2. Choi, C., Münch, R., Bunk, B., Barthelmes, J., Ebeling, C., Schomburg, D., Schobert, M., Jahn, D.: Combination of a data warehouse concept with web services for the establishment of the pseudomonas systems biology database systomonas. J. Integr. Bioinform. **4**(1), 12–21 (2007)

3. Capitani di Vimercati, S., Foresti, S., Livraga, G., Samarati, P.: Protecting privacy in data release. In: Aldini, A., Gorrieri, R. (eds.) FOSAD 2011. LNCS, vol. 6858, pp. 1–34. Springer, Heidelberg (2011). doi:10.1007/978-3-642-23082-0_1

4. Dwork, C.: Differential privacy. In: Bugliesi, M., Preneel, B., Sassone, V., Wegener, I. (eds.) ICALP 2006. LNCS, vol. 4052, pp. 1–12. Springer, Heidelberg (2006). doi:10. 1007/11787006_1

5. El Emam, K., Fineberg, A.: An overview of techniques for de-identifying personal health information. Access to Information and Privacy Division of Health Canada (2009)

6. Ferraiolo, D.F., Sandhu, R.S., Gavrila, S.I., Kuhn, D.R., Chandramouli, R.: Proposed NIST standard for role-based access control. ACM Trans. Inf. Syst. Secur. **4**(3), 224–274 (2001)

7. Garde, S., Hovenga, E.J.S., Buck, J., Knaup, P.: Ubiquitous information for ubiquitous computing: expressing clinical data sets with openEHR archetypes. In: MIE, pp. 215–220 (2006)

8. Kreger, H.: Web services conceptual architecture (WSCA 1.0). Technical report, IBM Software Group, May 2001

9. Liu, Z., Qamar, N., Qian, J.: A quantitative analysis of the performance and scalability of de-identification tools for medical data. In: Gibbons, J., MacCaull, W. (eds.) FHIES 2013. LNCS, vol. 8315, pp. 274–289. Springer, Heidelberg (2014). doi:10.1007/978-3-642-53956-5_18

10. McDonald, C.J., Blevins, L., Dexter, P.R., Schadow, G., Hook, J., Abernathy, G., Dugan, T., Martin, A., Phillips, D.R., Davis, M.: Demonstration of the Indianapolis SPIN query tool for de-identified access to content of the Indiana network for patient care's (a real RHIO) database. In: American Medical Informatics Association Annual Symposium (AMIA 2006), Washington, DC, USA, 11–15 November 2006 (2006)

11. Statistics Netherlands. u-argus user's manual. http://neon.vb.cbs.nl/casc/Software/MuManual4.2.pdf

12. Oster, S., Langella, S., Hastings, S., Ervin, D., Madduri, R.K., Phillips, J., Kurç, T.M., Siebenlist, F., Covitz, P.A., Shanbhag, K., Foster, I.T., Saltz, J.H.: Model formulation: cagrid 1.0: an enterprise grid infrastructure for biomedical research. JAMIA **15**(2), 138–149 (2008)

13. Ping, X.-O., Chung, Y., Tseng, Y.-J., Liang, J.-D., Yang, P.-M., Huang, G.-T., Lai, F.: A web-based data-querying tool based on ontology-driven methodology and flowchart-based model. JMIR Med. Inform. **1**(1), e2 (2013)

14. Prather, J.C., Lobach, D.F., Goodwin, L.K., Hales, J.W., Hage, M.L., Hammond, W.E.: Medical data mining: knowledge discovery in a clinical data warehouse. In: American Medical Informatics Association Annual Symposium (AMIA 1997), Nashville, TN, USA, 25–29 October 1997 (1997)

15. Price, M., Weber, J., McCallum, G.: Scoop - the social collaboratory for outcome oriented primary care. In: Proceedings of IEEE International Conference on Computer Based Medical Systems 27–29 May 2014 (2014)

16. Qamar, N., Faber, J., Ledru, Y., Liu, Z.: Automated reviewing of healthcare security policies. In: Weber, J., Perseil, I. (eds.) FHIES 2012. LNCS, vol. 7789, pp. 176–193. Springer, Heidelberg (2013). doi:10.1007/978-3-642-39088-3_12

17. Qamar, N., Ledru, Y., Idani, A.: Validation of security-design models using Z. In: Qin, S., Qiu, Z. (eds.) ICFEM 2011. LNCS, vol. 6991, pp. 259–274. Springer, Heidelberg (2011). doi:10.1007/978-3-642-24559-6_19

18. Samarati, P.: Protecting respondents' identities in microdata release. IEEE Trans. Knowl. Data Eng. **13**(6), 1010–1027 (2001)

19. Sweeney, L.: Simple demographics often identify people uniquely, pp. 50–59. Carnegie Mellon University, Pittsburgh, Data Privacy Working Paper 3 (2000)
20. Templ, M.: Statistical disclosure control for microdata using the R-package sdcMicro. Trans. Data Priv. **1**(2), 67–85 (2008)
21. Xiao, X., Wang, G., Gehrke, J.: Interactive anonymization of sensitive data. In: Proceedings of the ACM SIGMOD International Conference on Management of Data (SIGMOD 2009), pp. 1051–1054 (2009)

Author Index

Printed in the United States
By Bookmasters